CIVIL WAR
MEDICINE
1861–1865

Other books in the *Illustrated Living History Series*
by C. Keith Wilbur, M.D.

Pirates and Patriots of the Revolution

Revolutionary Medicine 1700–1800

Revolutionary Soldier

The New England Indians

Tall Ships of the World

Early Explorers of North America

Homebuilding and Woodworking in Colonial America

Indian Handcrafts

Woodland Indians

Illustrated Living History Series

CIVIL WAR
MEDICINE
1861–1865

by

C. Keith Wilbur, M.D.

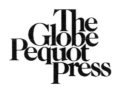

The
Globe
Pequot
Press

Old Saybrook, Connecticut

Cover design by Lana Mullen

Library of Congress Cataloging-in-Publication Data

Wilbur, C. Keith, 1923–
    Civil War medicine, 1861–1865 / by C. Keith Wilbur.
      p.   cm.   —(Illustrated living history series)
    Includes bibliographical references and index.
    ISBN 0-7627-0341-5
     1. United States—History—Civil War, 1861–1865—Medical care.
  2. Medicine, Military—United States—History—19th century.
  I. Title. II. Series: Wilbur, c. Keith, 1923– Illustrated living history series.
  E621.W56   1998
  973.7'75—dc21   98-30569
                                                           CIP

Manufactured in the United States of America
First Edition/First Printing

Contents

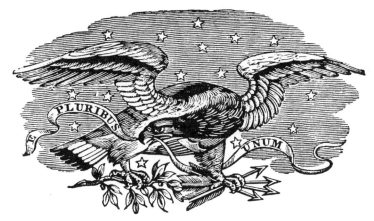

FOREWORD

I still remember as a boy reading about the death of the last Civil War veteran in our New England town. The obituary had been brief and businesslike, without answers to the questions that came to mind. What must it have been like to prepare for battle with only his convictions to help him face what might be his last minutes on earth? His bravery must have been riddled with fear as he made ready to charge the enemy's earthworks with his comrades. Facing a bristle of bayonets or exploding shells could easily exchange one's confidence for a buckling of the knees and a silent last-minute prayer.

Victory or retreat, the price must be a battlefield left with its scattering of the wounded and dying. The medical and surgical knowledge of those days had gradually geared up to meet such challenges never imagined in the yesterdays past. In the pages that follow, you'll read how outmoded theories hobbled the doctor, how surgeons soon became experts in the field hospitals, how women first entered a man's army as nurses, and how the civilian population joined together to show that prevention rather than treatment could save many of their soldiers' lives.

As I recall, our local Civil War veteran had been wounded and had likely undergone a battlefield rescue, taken a painful ambulance ride to the field hospital, and on to recovery at a general hospital. Since he can no longer describe his ordeals under the scalpel for us, Civil War Medicine 1861-1865 will have to do. May this book give a wider appreciation of the dedicated efforts of the Union and Confederate doctors and nurses to make each sick or wounded soldier whole again.

BEFORE SUMPTER

The 1856-57 teaching sessions at New York Medical College had ended. The student body had assembled to hear Dr. Timothy Childs's overview of the healing arts.

"In no period of the history of medicine has there been witnessed a progress at all comparable to that which has characterized the last quarter of a century. This was to be expected. Medicine can improve only as the collateral and tributary sciences improve — as these are perfected and applied to the study of our science, and as nature is more severely interrogated by better and more thorough methods of investigation. Medicine does improve, but it improves slowly."

If there was a touch of pride in the doctor's remarks it must be remembered that the American medical schools and the medicine they taught had made remarkable progress. It was only three-quarters of a century since the states had united to win their independence from the British Empire. No need to head overseas any longer for a better medical education — progress indeed. Still, there was an uneasiness in the air with all the secessionist saber-rattling going on. The possibility of war between these united states was not to be taken lightly. If put to the test, would the medical training offered on this side of the Atlantic be adequate to cope with such a disaster?

MEDICAL PROGRESS

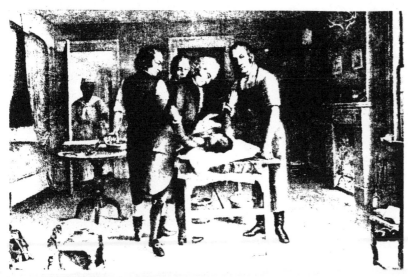

DR. McDOWELL'S KITCHEN OVARIOTOMY, DECEMBER, 1809

But on a more optimistic note, young America had not been standing idle over the operating table. In 1809 Dr. Ephraim McDowell of Danville, Kentucky, found himself in a no-win surgical dilemma. Jane Crawford's protruding abdomen hadn't yielded its expected twins and McDowell was called in consult for a house call some 60 miles away. The "pregnancy" turned out to be a 20-pound ovarian tumor.

Opening the abdomen in those presterilization days usually ended in death — but the result would be the same if the mass were not excised. Mrs. Crawford and her unwanted poundage made the trip on horseback to the doctor in the dead of winter. The kitchen table served as an operating table. Since anesthesia had yet to be discovered, the patient loudly sang hymns throughout the thirty minutes of surgery. They must have been heard by a higher power, for the lady lived on for thirty-one more years while McDowell took his place with the other pioneers of gynecological history.

Somehow Surgeon McDowell had invaded a body cavity without the almost inevitable "inflammation" spreading throughout the body to end in the death of its victim. As for his patient, singing hymns would have made a poor second to some kind of knockout anesthesia. Actually, there seemed promise of just such a surgical sleep in 1800 when nitrous oxide was

1

suggested as an anesthetic. It was an idea whose time hadn't yet arrived. Then in 1842, American surgeon Crawford W. Long gave a patient a few whiffs of ether vapor before excising a cystic neck tumor. Three years later he used the same anesthetic to deliver an infant. Unfortunately, Dr. Long hadn't made his successes public. Now his name is all but lost in a brief footnote to medical history.

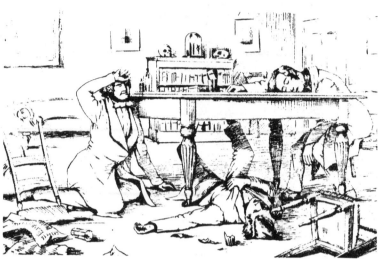

AN 1857 EXPERIMENT WITH CHLOROFORM

It was in 1844 that Dr. Horace Wells, a Hartford, Connecticut, dentist, was among the audience watching a "laughing gas" show. When a volunteer fell to the floor after inhaling the nitrous oxide gas, he felt no pain from his injured leg. Wells pondered what he had witnessed, and the next day he had the demonstrator give him the gas before having a dental student extract a bad molar. He was pain free. He hurried the news to a former dental partner, Dr. William Morton, who had moved to Boston. The doctor shared his excitement and obtained permission from Dr. John Collins Warren to demonstrate a pain-free tooth extraction. Supposedly anesthetized, the patient let out a scream when the forceps were applied. The students rocked the amphitheater with laughter instead of applause, and Wells retreated in disgrace to his home state.

Fortunately Morton shrugged off the failure and began to experiment with chloric ether. Here was another gas that made tooth extraction pain free, and he once again approached Warren for permission to test the new gas before witnesses. October 16, 1846, was the day that history was made in the Massachusetts General amphitheater— the same room where Wells's hopes had been shattered. After giving the patient a three-minute dose of the gas, Morton looked up and said to Warren, "Sir, your patient is ready." No doubt there was a collective holding of breath from the observers as the first scalpel cut was made. There were no screams this time ~ only silence as the surgeon removed the congenital vascular neck tumor. Warren then turned to the gallery and then made his enthusiastic pro-

MORTON'S INHALER

nouncement: "Gentlemen, this is no humbug!"

Morton's success was followed by a clincher the next day when he anesthetized another patient with a good-sized fatty shoulder tumor. On November 18, 1846, the prestigious "Boston Medical and Surgical Journal" announced surgery's great breakthrough to the rest of the world.

Horace Wells

INFLAMMATION THEORIES

When Professor Childs spoke to the students of New York Medical College about recent medical advances, pain-free surgery must have been one of the first to come to mind. But few if any who heard the talk and considered why medical progress had improved so slowly would suspect the faulty reasoning that had left the causes of infection undiscovered. Everyone knew that its symptoms of heat, redness, swelling, and pain could easily send a patient on a downhill course of gangrene and death. But who in the medical profession could even imagine microscopic germs invading the body through dirty wounds or being carried internally by tainted water or food? No, the inflammation theory was firmly implanted in every physician's practice and that was that.

Every medical student and graduate knew about Dr. William Cullen's mid-eighteenth-century assumption that the cause of inflammation was "nervous irritability." Another Edinburgh physician, Dr. John Brown, had gone one step further by theorizing that ANY excessive stimulation could cause overexcitement in one's body ~ otherwise known as inflammation.

DIRECT AND INDIRECT INFLAMMATION ~ Brown had recommended treating the body's excessive inflammatory excitement by relaxation. Bleeding, purgatives, narcotics, and counterirritants seemed reasonable treatments. But if a lack of stimulation left the body exhausted, the cure would include an overabundance of food, horseback riding, and massive doses of stimulating drugs.

Unfortunately, Brown's old theories (called Brunonian) unencumbered by facts, continued throughout the coming Civil War. By that time an updating had separated inflammation into direct and indirect subdivisions. Direct inflammation was caused by a blow, bullet, bayonet, burn, local irritant, or some such external stimuli. Usually treating these direct traumas would require the skills of a surgeon.

Indirect inflammation involved the internal organs of the body and were considered off limits to the surgeon. Opening any body cavity in the surgeon's unsterilized world was a sentence of death. Still, such organs had been studied under the microscope, and there was no doubt about their rich blood vessel and nerve supply. It was an easy next step to the theory that therefore each organ could be made easily irritated and hypersensitive with an excess of circulating blood (plethora). A ruddy complexion, then, was an outward sign that internal troubles were brewing. Immoderate food or drink, overexertion, exposure to bad air (mal-aria) from swamps or putrid matter, contact with cold air or water, disorders of the blood-purifying organs such as the liver, kidneys, and skin, or a debilitated state would push the patient into acute indirect inflammation.

The treatment for indirect inflammation was the practice of physick ~ that is, physicians using medicines instead of scalpels. Usually surgeons and physicians were one and the same doctor, but as the Civil War progressed, the doctors' duties became somewhat more specialized. Surgery would dominate in such "direct inflammation" centers as the field hospitals ~ the emergency first stop from the battlefield by way of an ambulance ~ to the military general hospitals where further surgical correction and "indirect inflammatory" medicines could be given in less urgent surroundings.

3

INDIRECT INFLAMMATORY TREATMENT

It seemed obvious that a physician must counter indirect inflammation by decreasing the amount of blood circulating in an inflamed organ, reducing any pain and nervous excitement, and removing any accumulated poisonous wastes by increased sweating, urination, and evacuation of the bowels. Not at all obvious were the unseen bacteria causing those inflammatory symptoms of heat, redness, swelling, and pain that could lead to gangrene and the last state of all: death.

BLEEDING~ Bleeding certainly did reduce excess circulation, a rapid pulse, and nervous excitement. Usually letting an average of 15 ounces of blood would do the trick and bring on the sought-after symptoms of a fluttering pulse, pallid lips, a blue-gray tint around the eyes, a decreased awareness of pain, and a relaxation that bordered on unconsciousness. Fortunately, voices were being raised against such a practice. The well-documented Effects of Bloodletting by Dr. Pierre Louis, published in 1835, was likely instrumental in reversing the trend. By the time of the Civil War, few if any soldiers were subjected to bleeding, leaving a full complement of white blood cells ready to do battle with any invasive bacteria.

SPRING LANCET

THE SCARIFICATOR MADE MULTIPLE GASHES IN THE SKIN AND BLED BY SUCTION CUPPING.

LEECHES!!

Constantly on hand a large stock of SWEDISH AND HUNGARIAN LEECHES of all sizes. Direct importation from his Breeding Ponds in Europe, always at the lowest European market prices.

Packages made up to insure a safe arrival for any country and climate. A prospectus describing the means of preserving them in a healthy state at all seasons of the year, together with a price list, sent by mail, free of expense, on application.

FOR SALE BY J. C. GALOUPEAU,
of late firm of C. PATUREL & Co.,
Importer of French Patent Medicines, India Rubber and Goat Skin Condoms, &c., and General Commission Merchant,

292 PEARL STREET, NEW YORK.

(House in Europe.)

N.B.—I would inform the trade that I keep none but the *very best* quality of *Medicinal Leeches,* and I will guarantee their superiority over all others in the market. 41.52

LEECHES PROVIDED THEIR OWN INCISING AND BLOOD SUCKING APPARATUS.

PURGATIVES ~ The mucous glands that lined the intestines could be stimulated by irritants, thereby flushing out any poisons believed to have caused organic inflammation. The preferred oral purgatives were calomel, colocynth, jalap, rhubarb, croton oil, sulphate of magnesia, and saline solutions. If the oral route left something to be desired, the other end could be pumped with such enemas as warm water or up to two pounds of gruel.

CATHARTICS ~ These intestinal scourers weren't all that different from the purgatives except that they were supposed to stimulate sluggish intestinal nerves leading to the body's filtering organs. The liver, pancreas, and intestines were thereby encouraged to pour out inflammatory poisons through the intestinal routes. Podophyllin was preferred over the poisonous mercury compound of calomel.

PEWTER AND HARD RUBBER CLYSTER ENEMAS

DIAPHORETICS ~ Inflammatory poisons could also be expelled through the sweat glands of the skin by increasing perspiration. Tartrate of antimony was favored over opium with ipecac (otherwise known as Dover's Powder). Warm baths would accompany the diaphoretic.

NARCOTICS ~ The symptoms of brain inflammation began with headaches, followed by dizziness, visual problems, restlessness, agitation, perhaps sleeplessness, illusions, and on to rigidity, paralysis, and coma. As with all infections, heat, redness, swelling, and pain were inevitable. Narcotics were given to relax the irritability present. Although opium could sometimes "lock up the bowels," it was more sleep-producing than its poisonous substitutes of henbane, hemlock, and the extracts of aconite and belladonna.

AMERICAN MEDICAL MONTHLY ADVERTISEMENT, 1858

COUNTERIRRITANTS ~ Inflammation of internal organs could be diluted and diffused by a competing skin irritant. The 1857 book Mitchell's Therapeutics put it this way: counterirritants were "the setting up of a new action in the neighborhood of a diseased spot with the view of transferring it from its original seat, as in the use of blisters for the relief of pleurisy." Blisters were produced on the overlying skin of the problem, and a plaster of "Spanish Fly" was a favorite. The irritating powder was of dried and crushed beetles, a sure-fire producer of skin bubbles. Each bleb would then be sliced open and more powder added to encourage drainage of the diseased serum.

There were other ways to inflict counterirritant misery on a patient. The more gentle these evils, known as rubefacients, were mustard, oil of turpentine, ammonia, gum ammoniac, camphor, and some of the mineral acids. Symes Surgery of 1857 took the no-nonsense approach with this recommendation: "when the effect is wishing to be strong and immediate, recourse may be had to boiling water"!

The Seton needle was the least endearing of the lot. A fold of skin near an internal inflammation site would be grasped and the lancelike needle driven through the doubled layers. A loosely woven silk or cotton tape was threaded through the eye of the needle and drawn through, leaving a length of wick on both sides of the punctured skin fold. A more permanent channel was the use of a red-hot cautery iron to sear through the drainage holes. Fortunately these more drastic counterirritants, like the practice of bleeding, had largely given way by the start of America's Civil War.

SETON NEEDLE

HERE, A SHARP-POINTED BISTOURY OPENED A SKIN FOLD TO PASS AN EYED PROBE. THE THREAD REMAINED IN PLACE.

AN UNSUNG HERO

Misconceptions, theories, and traditions had conspired against those who would soon be taking a part in preserving or severing the union of the American states. If ever there was a time for a keen mind and sharp eyes, this was it. A close second look at "laudable pus" under the microscope might question why all those minute dots and rods were engulfed in the phagocytic white blood cells. But then today's "retrospectoscope" can always bring the solutions to past problems clearly into focus. A century from now, our so-called modern medical miracles may raise more than a few eyebrows.

MICROSCOPIC PUS CELLS IN DRUITT'S MODERN SURGERY OF 1848 WITH "MINUTE GRANULES" THAT WERE PROBABLY UNRECOGNIZED BACTERIA

Yet back in those pre-Civil War days, there WAS a voice that dared question the authority of the theorists. Dr. Ignaz Philipp Semmelweiss joined the obstetrical staff of Vienna Krankenhous after his medical school graduation. At the end of his first year, he was distressed to count no less than 451 mothers who had died on the staff ward of puerperal (childbearing) fever within a week of delivery. Surprisingly, on a ward staffed only by midwives, the "childbed fever" cases numbered a modest 90 deaths.

An important piece of the puzzle fell into place when the ward pathologist cut himself during an autopsy and died of "inflammation." Semmelweiss realized that the pathologist's skin lesions were identical to those of patients who had died of puerperal fever ~ AND that its carriers were the ward obstetrical doctors who routinely attended the morning autopsies before going on rounds to examine the recently delivered women. It seemed clear that some invisible inflammatory poison had been carried from the puerperal fever victims. Semmelweiss made no friends when he insisted that the wards be scrubbed clean with calcium chloride and that every doctor wash his hands thoroughly before examining or delivering any maternity patient. Within two years the ward death rate plummeted to almost nothing.

When Semmelweiss presented his findings to the Vienna Medical Society, he was roundly ridiculed. Not to be outdone, the hospital dismissed him from the staff ~ and the maternity ward deaths soared to their old highs. The medical community just couldn't come to grips with a concept so much at odds with the honored inflammation theory. Semmelweiss would not be stilled. After being chosen as professor of obstetrics at Budapest University in 1855, he published his famous treatise on "The Cause, Concept, and Prophylaxis of Puerperal Fever" in 1861, the same year that the Northern and Southern states clashed in an all-out Civil War.

OBSTETRIC POUCH

One might wonder why the germ theory was so difficult to accept when microscopes had become more widely available during the first half of the nineteenth century. Actually it was almost impossible to spot a one-celled troublemaker amid the cells of the body without a culture or a specific stain ~ and, of course, an inquisitive mind to consider what mischief might be hidden in all that protoplasm. That questioning mind would arrive one day in the person of Louis Pasteur. But his discoveries twenty years after the Civil War were much too late to help the thousands of soldiers who stopped a bullet or fell victim to one of the contagious diseases.

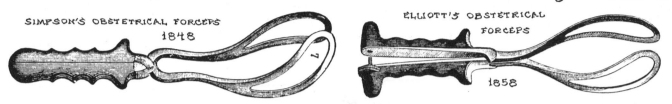

SIMPSON'S OBSTETRICAL FORCERS 1848

ELLIOTT'S OBSTETRICAL FORCEPS

1858

HARD LESSONS FROM CRIMEA 1854-56

A preview of the soon-to-come American Civil War was being fought on the Crimean Peninsula. There a beleaguered Turkey and her English, French, and Sardinian allies were pitted against Russian troops intent on laying siege to Constantinople and winning a direct outlet to the Mediterranean Sea. Still alive in every general's mindset was that a battlefield's dead and dying were handicaps to a sustained offensive. The business of war must move ahead. Perhaps the casualties could be removed in a few days when the enemy had been routed. Any relief would be in the form of a makeshift hospital filled with closely packed bodies. There dysentery or cholera might well finish what a bullet failed to do.

Into those woeful conditions sailed a team of thirty-eight English nurses, headed by a very capable Nurse Florence Nightingale and sent by the British Sanitary Commission. This was the first time that English women had ever staffed a military hospital, for women were generally considered delicate homemakers and not a part of the rough-and-tumble business of warfare. The contingent arrived at the hospital just as did a crush of 500 wounded British soldiers. They were in desperate shape, for they had lain on the Balaklava battlefield for ten days ~ unwashed, without bandages for their wounds, in pain, and without food.

Nightingale moved quickly to have brought ashore the stalled shiploads of medical supplies, cots, and mattresses into the wards. Both the wards and the men who filled them were scrubbed down, and fresh, nourishing meals were brought to the half-starved soldiers. Nurse Nightingale's ongoing sanitation measures soon reduced the ward death toll from the usual 42 percent to 2 percent. Even so, one medical army supervisor cautioned her "not to spoil the brutes"!

Dr. Semmelweiss had given notice of contagious inflammatory poisons to a world not yet ready to discard the old theories of disease. But

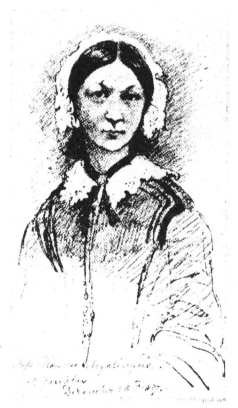

FLORENCE NIGHTINGALE IN 1857
PENCIL DRAWING BY SIR GEORGE SCHARF

...ingale had underlined the value of such simple and reason-
...ighting measures as cleanliness, fresh and wholesome food
...bedding, and light and airy surroundings. There was abun-
... such measures, supervised by a dedicated and knowl-
...staff, could greatly reduce the warfare deaths from
...nds. For now and until the bacterial cause for infection
...s proved, proper sanitation in every camp or on every battlefield would do more to preserve life than would most surgical procedures
or any quantity of medicine. But would the Union or Confederate surgeon
generals be paying attention?

THAT CHAOTIC FIRST YEAR

The bombardment of Fort Sumpter had announced, loud and clear, that peace between the states had been wishful thinking. At least it shouldn't take long to punish the Rebels— or the "damnyankees"— for their misguided notions. President Lincoln called on the North- ern states to provide 75,000 state militiamen for a three-month enlistment. Patriotism had reached a fever pitch. On Volunteer Days in both North and South, the flag-draped village squares, music from the local band, an army officer in dress uniform, and pretty girls in plenty could fill the town's quota of volunteers in less than an hour. They would be enlisted directly into the Federal or the Confederate service.

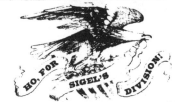

But quantity had no bearing on quality. Some states did give fairly thorough strip-down physical examinations similar to those given to a career enlistee. Others offered little more than a thump on the chest and a few knee and elbow flexes — a quick fix for a short-term duty. Some 400 women passed through the examinations undetected and served in the Union ranks!

Dr. A. J. Phelps, in his "Sanitary Memoirs of the War," wrote that "feeble boys, toothless old men, consumptives, asthmatics, one-eyed, one-armed men, men with different length of legs, club-footed and ruptured, and, in short, men with every variety of disability, and whose systems were replete with the elements of disease were accepted as recruits and started to the field only to become a tax upon the government and to encumber the movements of its armies." The Union Army of the Potomac finally discharged soldiers at a rate of nearly three who were handicapped before enlistment for every soldier disabled for wounds or disease while on active duty.

In Rebel country it wasn't until the fall of 1862 that physical examination guidelines were issued by Medical Department authorities. Even then such problems as partial deafness, reducible hernias, blindness in one eye, or the loss of several fingers were acceptable for active duty. The Confederacy also discovered through experience that men of the age of forty or older were sure targets for diseases and deaths from the strain and contacts of camp life.

THE MEDICAL DEPARTMENTS

The United States Army had been resting on its laurels. The American Revolution, the War of 1812, the recent Mexican War, and the occasional skirmishes with Indian uprisings were all in the win column. Now only a token force of 16,000 soldiers was scattered over the countryscape to keep the peace. Army life was a prestigious life with few demands or need for updating the art of warfare. Many officers were veterans of the War of 1812 with Britain, a roster of deadwood that enjoyed seniority promotions that knew no age or disability requirements. The rumblings of Southern discontent sounded more like taps than reveille to the old-timers in the various departments of the army.

A case in point was the United States Army Medical Department, where Surgeon General Dr. Thomas Lawson marked time in his declining years. Well into his eighties, Lawson's goal in life seemed to be one of slashing his Medical Department ex-

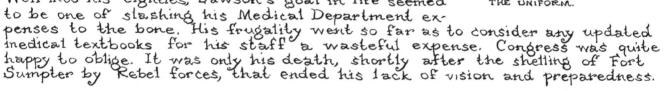

THE COAT OF ARMS OF THE MEDICAL DEPARTMENT WAS ADOPTED ABOUT 1818 AND IS THE OLDEST EMBLEM IN THE ARMY. IT WAS NOT WORN ON THE UNIFORM.

penses to the bone. His frugality went so far as to consider any updated medical textbooks for his staff a wasteful expense. Congress was quite happy to oblige. It was only his death, shortly after the shelling of Fort Sumpter by Rebel forces, that ended his lack of vision and preparedness.

Another War of 1812 veteran was next in line for the job. Handsome and with a military bearing that belied his years, Dr. Clement A. Finley turned out to be another shortsighted surgeon general. Since he considered any conflict with the Southern states a matter of short duration, there was no need for a costly buildup of Medical Department personnel. His peacetime mini-staff of thirty surgeons and the eighty-three assistant surgeons ~ usually fresh from medical school ~ could carry on as usual. Well, not quite. Eight of the surgeons and twenty-nine assistant surgeons would soon be resigning their commissions and following their sympathies to the Confederate Army. No matter, for the Northern medical schools were considered the best in the nation and could fill any gap that a civil unpleasantness might bring.

Dr. Samuel Preston Moore was the newly appointed Confederate surgeon general. Although he was also of a mind that an extended conflict was highly unlikely, haste must be made to staff the army Medical Department. Fortunately he had inherited none of the sluggish

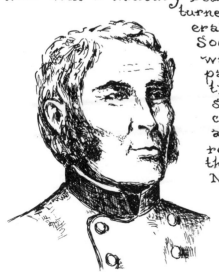

CONFEDERATE SURGEON GENERAL
SAMUEL MOORE (CONJECTURAL)

senility that plagued his Northern counterpart. By requiring screening examinations for all staff applicants, he was able to sidestep any politically appointed incompetents. One early disappointment must have been the Confederate Congress's shortsighted vote of but $50,000 to establish AND run all of the military hospitals throughout the South. Even so, Moore was determined to make his general hospitals state of the art throughout the war years.

ARMY DOCTORS OF VARIED ABILITIES

THE REGULARS ~ A backward glance at the medical training available in America is in order. The Regulars were the more highly regarded physicians who had graduated from medical school. While such prestigious schools as Harvard, Yale, Columbia, Princeton, and the University of Pennsylvania had been producing doctors since the eighteen century, the fifty years before the Civil War produced at least one new school a year. In the South, quality medical schools were to be found in Virginia, South Carolina, and Louisiana. Many others gave decent instruction, while others were fly-by-night affairs of poor quality. Unfortunately there were no standards for receiving an M.D. degree.

New England did spearhead a drive for uniform quality of medical training, and in 1847 the American Medical Association came into being for that purpose. It wasn't until as late as 1912 that the Federation of State Medical Boards finally provided America's guidelines for improving medical education and standardizing state licenses for the practice of medicine. Until then, all that was needed to constitute a medical school were several doctors giving a series of lectures under some sort of roofing that could ward off inclement weather.

Admit C. G. King (TO THE) Massachusetts General Hospital. Boston 1855

Harvard University. LECTURES ON Anatomy & Physiology BY O. W. HOLMES M.D. Admit C. G. Carleton 1863

ADMISSION CARDS FOR MEDICAL SCHOOL LECTURES AND HOSPITAL ROUNDS

No. 297 Nov 1845 UNIVERSITY OF Pennsylvania LECTURES ON THE Principles & Practice of SURGERY BY William Gibson, M.D. For Mr. J. G. Parkinson

Large or small, every medical school usually lacked hands-on contact with live patients ~ or cadavers for anatomical dissection for that matter. In 1830, Massachusetts recognized the need for its future doctors to learn anatomy from real flesh and blood and made it legal for medical schools to accept bodies for that purpose. Very few other states followed suit before the Civil War. Grave robbing, despite the threat of imprisonment and an angry public, still took place in the dark shadows of local cemeteries.

John Brown's 1859 raid on Harper's Ferry offered a possible source. After Brown and his followers did battle with Federal troops, commanded by none other than Colonel Robert E. Lee, it occurred to the students of Winchester Medical College of Virginia that a spare body might have been left behind. Every student in school boarded the train for that battle site and did indeed find one of the undiscovered dead. After the corpse was shipped back to the school, papers were found on it that identified the body as John Brown's son, Owen. Many Northerners considered Brown's raid a heroic adventure ~ even if ill advised. When Union troops captured the town of Winchester in 1862, their commander learned of the body-knapping and rescued the dry-prepared remains of Owen Brown. The college buildings were then burned to the ground in reprisal.

THE DOCTOR'S APPRENTICE ~ Since colonial times, apprenticeship had been a workable and less expensive alternative to medical school. A young man of fifteen or so years, with about a hundred dollars in his pocket to pay for a single year's instruction, would have access to the doctor's books, join him on his daily rounds, and assist in office surgery. His room and board would be included in the price. Since this was a work-learn experience, the student was expected to clean the office, run errands, water the horses, compound and dispense medications, and any other chores at hand. After a stint of between two and five years, the young doctor would face the competition for patients from the diploma mills or the Irregulars.

THE IRREGULARS ~ These were the medical mavericks who ran counter to the generally accepted medical thought. HOMEOPATHS gave infinitesimal amounts that if given in massive doses would produce symptoms similar to those being treated. ALLOPATHS used medicines that gave the opposite symptoms to those being treated. THE ECLECTICS straddled the fence and chose whatever theories they considered best from the broad spectrum of medical practice. Meanwhile the THOMSONIANS zeroed in on remedies that could be produced only from plants. HYDROPATHS were dedicated to drowning a disease with quantities of mineral water given both internally and externally.

This hodgepodge of medical practitioners ~ the Regulars, the Doctor's Apprentices, and the Irregulars ~ all with varied knowledge, beliefs, skills, and

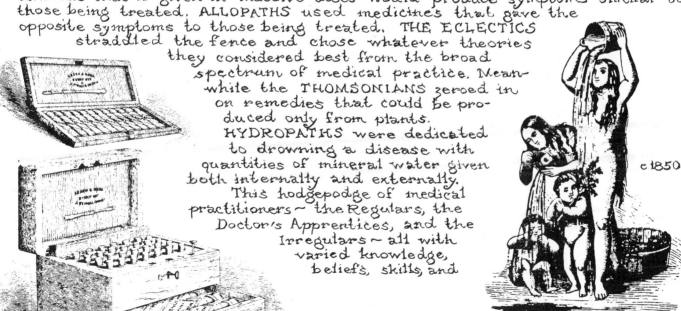

HOMEOPATHIC POCKET AND CASED MEDICINES, 1861

c 1850

WATER, WATER EVERYWHERE FOR WATER CURE ENTHUSIASTS

experience, would now be asked to do what they could for the overwhelming numbers of sick and wounded Civil War casualties. At best, the outlook seemed mighty discouraging.

When a Northern or Southern state had assembled enough men to reach a regimental strength of 1,200 volunteers, Congress authorized the governor of that state to appoint a regimental surgeon and an assistant surgeon. They must first pass a medical competency review by a Medical Examining Board. In reality most of these regimental doctors were chosen by the senior regimental officer; a judgment that had little bearing on competency.

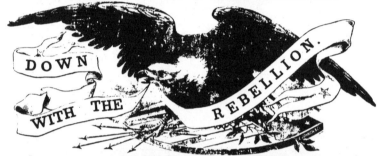

FOURTH REGIMENT
NEW HAMPSHIRE

DOWN WITH THE REBELLION.

VOLUNTEERS.

ABLE BODIED MEN WANTED
FOR THE FOURTH REGIMENT.

The subscribers having been appointed Recruiting Officers, will open a Recruiting Office at

Where they will enlist all who would like to rally around the OLD STARS AND STRIPES, the emblem of America's Freedom.

$10 BOUNTY WILL BE ALLOWED!
Regular Army pay and Rations to commence on taking the oath.

Lieut. J. M. CLOUGH,
Sergt. W. B. ROWE.

Sept. 1861.

Repr. Holley & Co., Printers

THE REGIMENTAL TRADITION

In days past, when wars on American soil were relatively small in scale, individual regiments functioned as small armies within an army. Any emergency increase in regular army manpower would be in the form of volunteer regiments supplied through each state's quota. States' rights were jealously guarded, and a call for state assistance did provide a check on any excessive Federal military power. The downside was a state regiment officered by nonprofessionals of varied abilities. And so it was with each state-appointed regimental surgeon and assistant surgeon, for their backgrounds and experience often had little in common.

Each Union and Confederate state-supplied surgeon and his assistant~ usually a doctor fresh out of medical school~had a hospital steward and between ten and twelve noncombatants as aids. These untrained helpers were convalescent or otherwise incapacitated soldiers and perhaps the regiment's band members who had no place in battle. Until the volunteer regiments supplied by the states had built up combat strength, the three tents assigned to each regimental campsite hosted the usual camp diseases, a blister here or a cut there.

Once the volunteer regiment marched into battle, the true mettle of its doctors was revealed. As soon as the troops were positioned on the battlefield, the assistant surgeon, his

CONFEDERATE STATES

MEDICAL & SURGICAL

EXPERIENTIA DOCET.

JOURNAL.

Vol. 1   RICHMOND, MARCH, 1864   No. 3

THIS JOURNAL WAS PUBLISHED BETWEEN JANUARY 1864 TO MARCH 1865 TO UPDATE THE CONFEDERATE ARMY DOCTORS.

hospital steward, and several helpers searched out a sheltered spot or perhaps a building within a few hundred yards of the front line. This would be the regimental emergency-aid ambulance depot where a red flag would be raised as a mustering guide for any of their wounded.

Those who could move under their own power would walk, while the more severely injured would be carried in on stretchers by the helpers. Assistant surgeons would control any hemorrhages, splint fractures, give pain medication, and perform any such first aid as was necessary before sending the casualties on to the surgeon at the regimental field hospital by ambulance. If all had gone well, the three tents or an abandoned building would serve as a shelter after amputations, trephinations, removal of bullets, stitching lacerations, and like surgery. While most would remain to recuperate in the regimental camp, the most severe cases might be brought to a makeshift general military hospital by ambulance for further observation or surgery.

All this seemed organized and efficient on paper, but each regiment was on its own, entirely dependent on its surgeon's skill and organizational ability. Some regiments might suffer heavy casualties that overwhelmed their field hospitals, while others might not see much or any action with little to be done in the way of surgery. Some surgeons might even refuse to accept casualties from the other harder-hit units. Each was an island unto itself with little or no direction or coordination from its surgeon general.

The great majority of regimental doctors were surgeons in name only. In civilian practice back home, the chance to practice surgery came so rarely that some young doctors enlisted as a patriotic way to become expert in the art. There was more than enough practice when the flood of casualties engulfed the regimental field hospital. There the primary amputations, within twenty-four hours of being wounded, would take place.

POCKET INSTRUMENT CASE NOTES

Regimental surgeons would have been well advised to carry the light pocket instrument case into service. For the most part the various blades were folded jackknife fashion into tortoise shell handles to save space and protect the cutting edges.

1-5 Scalpels were for incisions and dissections. Bistouries, named for a town called Pistori where many were made, had long narrow blades that were straight or curved with sharp or blunt (probe-pointed) tips. A straight sharp-pointed blade made precise incisions. A straight blunt-pointed blade could cut near deep arteries, nerves, and organs to prevent punctures. Curved sharp-pointed blades incised tissues with a grooved director, drained abscesses and collections of fluids, and opened sinuses and fistulas. This was probably the most-used blade. Curved blunt-pointed blades released strangulated hernia strictures and divided tendons.

6 Gum lancet—the tenaculum hooked and tied severed arteries.

7 Splinter forceps.

8 Artery forceps gripped the artery with grooved points or teeth and were held in place with a sliding or a spring catch. Another much used artery forceps had crossed arms that gripped firmly when the thumb pressure was released. In any case, a ligature with an overhand knot could be slipped down the forceps and around the artery for tying.

9 Liston's toothed forceps.

10-12 Angular scissors, guided along a grooved director, divided tissues, layed open fistulas, and removed roller bandages. Curved blades excised skin lesions and were useful when operating in bodily cavities. Straight scissors cut bandages and dressings.

13 Dressing forceps.

14 Caustic holder for a silver nitrate stick.

15 Probe with eye (see page 5 for its use as a seton needle).

16 Spatula with elevator for spreading plasters.

17 Grooved director with tongue tie for cutting tongue frenulum.

18 Vaccinator comb scarificator and lancet.

19 Abscess lancet.

20 Vaccinator with a groove in the blade to flow the vaccine under the pricked epidermis.

21 Thumb lancet for bleeding~rarely used after 1860.

22 Suturing needles.

23 Wooden or ivory suture frame held wound saddler's silk and iron, lead, and silver wire.

24 Finger saw for amputations.

25 Exploring needle with screw-in container handle removed tissue specimens for examination.

26 Male and female silver catheters were carried in sections.

CIVIL WAR POCKET CASE INSTRUMENTS

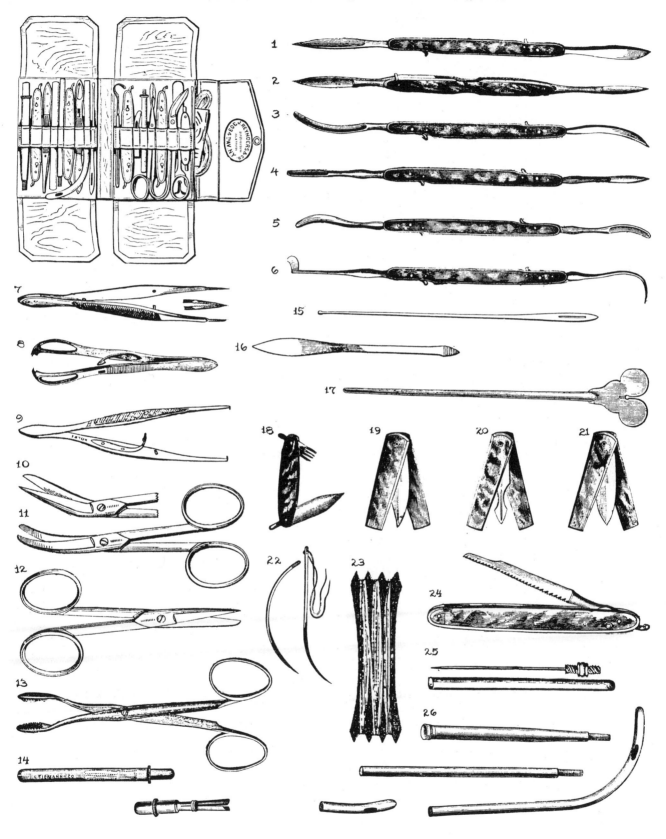

Likely many regimental surgeons could relate to Dr. Simon Baruch's experience under Stonewall Jackson's command. "I have never lanced a boil. At Second Manassas, a busy surgeon offered me a knife, saying, 'Doctor, perhaps you would like to operate?' I accepted the challenge. This was my first surgical operation of any kind. The surgeon was kind enough to commend my work."

Experience seemed the best teacher. Assistant Surgeon S.H. Melcher of the 5th Missouri Volunteers was on his own when battlefield casualties had infested wounds in the heat of the August 1861 sun. Later he wrote:

"The flies were exceedingly troublesome after the battle, maggots forming in the wounds in less than an hour after dressing them, and also upon any clothing or bedding soiled by blood or pus. The wounded left on the field in the enemy's hands were swarming with maggots when brought in. After several ineffectual attempts to extirpate these pests, I succeeded perfectly by sprinkling calomel freely over the wounded surface. When the sloughs separated, clean granulating surfaces were presented, and by using balsam of [copaiba] as a dressing, smearing the bandages with this oleoresin, I could keep the wounds free of maggots."

The relative isolation of every regimental surgeon could also bring on an acute shortage of medications. In the Union army, it was the practice of Surgeon General Finley to send along periodic allotments. A sudden camp epidemic of some disease, an unexpected battle in the offing, or just a surgeon's inexperience at proportioning medicine over such a large number of men could leave supplies at a dangerously low level. Even if Finley's generally slow response to such emergency battlefield drug needs were answered in a more timely manner, they might well be delayed or sidetracked by the higher priority munitions being hurried to the front.

The United States Sanitary Commission could be counted upon to come through in such a crisis situation. Many were the surgeons who depended on the Commission sidestepping governmental red tape and delivering needed chloroform, morphine, stimulants, dressings, and sponges to the front lines. At Antietam the Commission's agent reported

"within a week we dispatched by teams from Washington alone 28,700 shirts, drawers, blankets, bedticks, 30 barrels of bandages, 3000 pounds of farina, 2,600 pounds of condensed milk, 5,000 pounds of beef stock and canned meats, 3,600 bottles wine, and several tons of lemons and other fruits, crackers, tea, sugar, and other hospital conveniences."

Of all the regimental shortcomings, none were greater than the inefficient removal and treatment of the battlefield wounded. Not until well into the second year of the Civil War would the Union develop its outstanding ambulance recovery plan that would hurry the wounded to field hospitals where skilled surgical teams stood ready. Recuperation would take place in newly built general hospitals that did credit to both the Union and Confederate army medical departments. Meanwhile, the United States Sanitary Commission continued to preach the importance of maintaining the health and welfare of its Union troops.

THE UNITED STATES SANITARY COMMISSION

Somehow the very title "Sanitary Commission" sounded wimpy and ineffectual in an America that now reverberated with cannon and small arms fire, patriotic speeches, and long columns of soldiers marching into battle to the cadence of martial music. Perhaps so, but the women they left behind were determined to do their best to help their fighting men. It didn't matter that they might be considered meddlesome females. The United States Sanitary Commission became a reality through their backing and persistence. In a day when medicine was based largely on theoretical ideas, the Commission's emphasis on prevention rather than cure could save the lives of countless Union soldiers.

Briefly, it came about this way. In the North, Ladies Aid Societies blossomed everywhere until their sisterhoods numbered well over 7,000 strong. Mothers, wives, and sweethearts collected and sent articles of comfort and supplies of necessity to their boys in blue. But without some sort of representation to coodinate the effort between the many societies and the army ~ particularly the medical department ~ duplication and poor distribution would result. Four prominent citizens

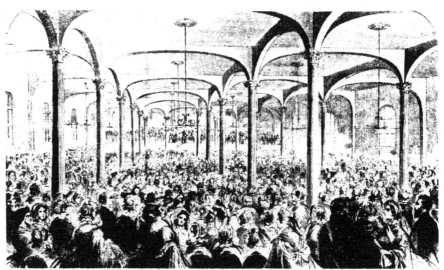

MEETING AT COOPER UNION HALL IN NEW YORK, APRIL 25, 1861, TO ORGANIZE THE WOMEN'S CENTRAL ASSOCIATION OF RELIEF

stepped forward to fill this leadership role: Dr. Henry Bellows, minister of All Souls Unitarian Church of New York; Dr. W. H. Van Buren, representing the Physicians and Surgeons of New York Hospital; Dr. Elisha Harris of the Women's Central Association; and Dr. Jacob Harsen of the Lint and Bandage Association.

By May 15, 1861, the four committeemen were on a train and Washington bound. As they talked of their mission, the possibility of a sanitary commission came to mind, perhaps using the successful British Sanitary Commission's blueprint. Certainly the Ladies Aid Societies were concerned with the health and welfare of their volunteer soldiers. But for any input clout, the proposed Commission must be an official arm of the Union war effort. The four committeemen found their reception less than enthusiastic.

Undismayed, the quartet bent many an ear in Washington's official circles. Patience and persistence were rewarded June 9 when a dubious President Lincoln signed the order creating the United States Sanitary Commission. He had been concerned that this home-front effort might be "a fifth wheel to the coach" ~ but the wave of enthusiasm that had engulfed all those well-meaning women would surely peter out in time. As for crusty old Surgeon General Finley, he believed that civilian do-gooders, including their volunteer soldiers, and their Commission deserved one another. Let the Com-

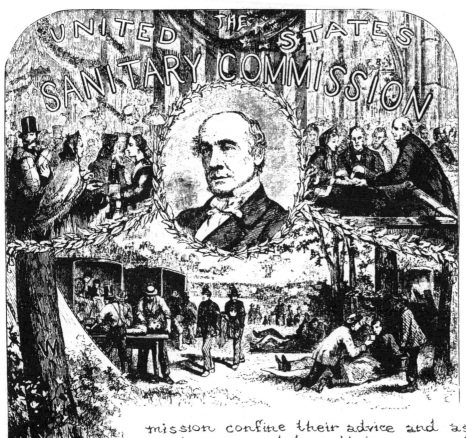

mission confine their advice and assistance to the volunteer servicemen, and keep their noses out of the tiny core of regular army personnel.

Essentially, the Commission now had the responsibility and power to investigate and recommend any sanitary reforms needed for practically all of the Union Army.

The nine civilian commissioners and the three army officers (who would supposedly act as a balance but who were usually away on other wartime duties) then made a most fortunate choice for their executive secretary. Frederick Law Olmsted, otherwise known as F.L.D., seemed at first glance to be an unlikely driving force for the Commission. He was crowding forty, was housed in a short, slight frame that carried a limp, wasn't in the best of health, and seemed better suited for continuing his well-known architectural designs and work force management in the building of New York's Central Park. But he was an unstoppable bulldog when it came to organization, leadership concentration, determining priorities, and a desire to better the human existence.

It was inevitable that Olmsted lock horns with the small-minded surgeon general. Just before the Battle of Bull Run, Commission inspection teams had found the sanitary conditions in the volunteer camps a disaster waiting to happen. Further, capable cooks and plenty of fresh vegetables were needed to improve the soldiers' health. These recommendations were defeated by the Senate

FREDERICK LAW OLMSTED

18

Military Affairs Committee for fear of any embarrassment to Surgeon General Finley.

REALITY AT BULL RUN

Union Field Nurse Emma Edmonds described Bull Run this way:

"Still the battle continues without cessation; the grape and canister fill the air as they go screaming on their fearful errand; the sight of that field is perfectly appalling; men tossing their arms wildly calling for help; they be bleeding, torn and mangled; legs, arms and bodies are crushed and broken as if smitten by thunderbolts; the ground is crimson with blood; it is terrible to witness."

The devastation looked no better through Rebel eyes. Medical Steward E. A. Craighill of Jackson's Brigade wrote on July 21, 1861:

"From at first we had nothing to do, it was not long before I had more than I could possibly do, because on the bloody field, very soon the wounded needed all my attention and until late into the night on that eventful day, my every minute was occupied with the dead and wounded."

Craighill went on to say, "Of course, there are surgeons in our army older than I was, who had much more experience, but none of us up to that time had seen much of gunshot wounds, and we had to unlearn what we had been taught in college in books as almost worthless, and only experience was useful in treatment and forming a correct or even an appropriate opinion of results from wounds particularly and sometimes from disease."

Here was the wake-up call, louder than a thousand bugles, for the surgeon generals of the opposing armies. Here was the first battlefield example of what this all-out war would be like. Basically, two armed mobs, undertrained and overconfident, had paid a high price in dead and wounded. The Southern forces had won the field and therefore had more leisure to give emergency care and removal of their fallen soldiers.

On the other hand, the Union retreat was confusion at its worst. When the dash back to the relative safety of Washington began, the civilian-driven empty ambulances and wagons all but led the way. Inexperienced regimental surgeons were left on their own with an impossible collection of hemorrhages, compound fractures and severe gunshot wounds. Those surgeons who remained on the Bull Run battlefield were taken prisoner, separated from

ON THE INNER LID:
"MEDICAL SCALES-
FOUND IN THE POCKET
OF A FEDERAL MEDICAL
OFFICER AFTER THE
BATTLE- BULL RUN - HE
BEING ONE OF THE DEAD."

GETTYSBURG NATIONAL MILITARY PARK

19

their patients, and transported to Richmond. The United States Commission, at least, was well into pressuring Surgeon General Finley into some sort of action, giving the civilians back home some hope and direction in the face of the Bull Run disaster and providing better long-term food, clothing, shelter, and cleanliness of both camp and person for every Union soldier. Olmsted had underlined the Commission's basic objective as "prevention rather than cure."

EVEN THE SCHOOL CHILDREN WERE DOING WHAT THEY COULD TO RAISE FUNDS THROUGH FAIRS, PLAYS, AND CONCERTS FOR THE UNITED STATES SANITARY COMMISSION'S GOALS.

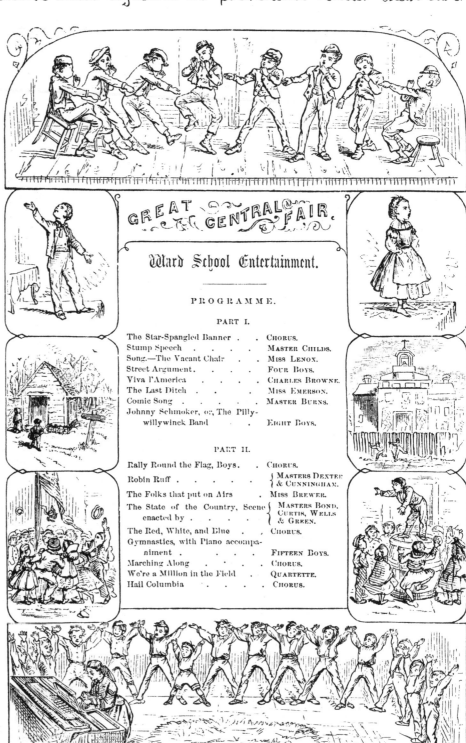

RATIONS

Federal and Confederate regulations endorsed the same daily ration allotments for the soldiers under arms.

1. Salt pork~ one ration was 12 ounces, one hundred rations (a company) was 125 pounds. This was the principal meat ration. On the march, it might be eaten uncooked with hardtack but was better disguised in soups or lobscouse. When served in the company kitchen, it was usually boiled.

2. Fresh beef (in place of salt beef) ~ one ration was 20 ounces, one hundred rations 125 pounds. Because little water was available on the march, the beef was reserved for a more settled camp life. Since the Confederates had little salt or other preservatives for their meat, much was lost from spoilage.

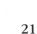

AN ARMY OVEN

3. Flour or fresh loaf bread ~ one ration was 18 ounces or if it was made of corn meal 20 ounces, one hundred rations was 112.5 pounds. For a time in 1861, the vaults under the western side of the capital were converted into bakeries. Sixteen thousand loaves were baked there each day. Surprisingly, the Union troops tired of it sooner than hard bread. For the Rebels, corn bread was made of coarse, unsifted meal, and their troops soon tired of its frequent servings.

4. Hard bread (hardtack) ~ one ration was 12 ounces, increased to 1 pound on the march, one hundred rations was 75 pounds. If boxed too soon after baking or if weather-dampened, the hard bread could become moldy. Maggots and weevils could be eliminated by crumbling into hot coffee and then skimmed off the surface. Confederates liked their hardtack soaked in bacon grease and fried; or on the march, a piece of fat pork with dry crackers.

FRYING HARDTACK

5. Potatoes ~ when practicable, one hundred rations was half a bushel.

6. Beans or peas ~ one hundred rations was 8 quarts or 15 pounds. In a settled camp, the company cooks stewed the beans with pieces of salt pork. On the march, six soldiers would often pool their rations and cook beanhole bean style ~ the most appreciated meal in the Union army. General Robert E. Lee was in agreement, for he called field peas the Confederate soldier's best friend.

7. Rice or hominy ~ one hundred rations was 10 pounds.

SOFT BREAD

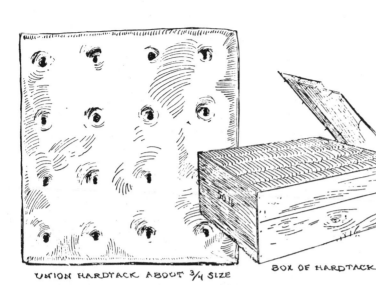

UNION HARDTACK ABOUT 3/4 SIZE

BOX OF HARDTACK

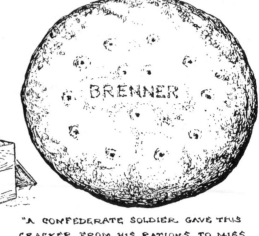

"A CONFEDERATE SOLDIER GAVE THIS CRACKER FROM HIS RATIONS TO MISS GOLDSBOROUGH OF SUMMIT POINT, WEST VIRGINIA, IN 1864. SHE KEPT IT AS A MOMENTO THROUGHOUT HER LIFE."
GETTYSBURG NATIONAL MILITARY PARK

8. Coffee— if green, one hundred rations was 10 pounds; if roasted and ground, one hundred rations was 8 pounds. If tea instead— one hundred rations was 24 ounces. Union coffee was generally of good quality and almost invariably used as a pick-me-up after a hard march or battle. For ease in carrying rations in the haversack on a march, the Yankee troops often mixed their coffee and sugar rations together. Condensed milk could be bought from the sutler if a soldier had enough jingle in his pockets.

As of January 1862 the Confederacy was no longer able to supply its soldiers with coffee. The brew was sorely missed, and many were the trial-and-error substitutes that followed. According to The Life of Johnny Reb, "an amber fluid was optimistically brewed from parched peanuts, potatoes, peas, dried apples, corn or rye. 'Tea' was made of corn, bran, ginger and herbs of various sorts. Sassafras tea was drunk in large quantities by privates and generals alike."

9. Vinegar— one hundred rations was one gallon.

10. Salt— one hundred rations was 2 quarts.

11. Sugar— one hundred rations was 15 pounds.

12. Molasses— one hundred rations was 1 quart. Southern troops couldn't obtain it but found sorghum a worthwhile substitute.

13. Pepper— one hundred rations was 4 ounces.

Although the above rations were considered a practical diet for a mid-nineteenth-century soldier, time has shown that it was anything but well rounded. Milk, leafy greens, yellow vegetables, and fruits were generally among the missing— along with the vitamins and minerals they supplied. Deficiency diseases were bound to surface, for garden-fresh produce were often out of season and

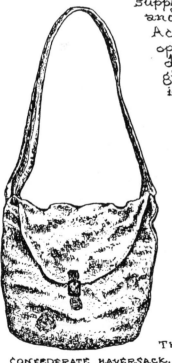

THIS CONFEDERATE HAVERSACK, USUALLY OF LINEN WITHOUT WATERPROOFING, CARRIED THE SOLDIER'S FOOD RATIONS
GETTYSBURG NATIONAL MILITARY PARK

perishable in transport.

The Union Commissary came up with an interesting solution and named it desiccated vegetables ~ otherwise known by the troops as "desecrated vegetables." An ounce ration of layered carrots, turnips, parsnips, leafy greens, and whatever else could be dried was squeezed into a cube. Soaking then swelled the cubed collection to several times its compressed size. Although it may have had the same taste appeal as wet cardboard, it was quite tolerable in soup. Unfortunately, any vitamin A was destroyed by drying and vitamin C by storage

The United States Sanitary Commission had taken notice of the dramatic health improvement when experienced English cooks were sent to their Crimean troops. As early as July 1861 they also sent knowledgeable cooks into more settled Union camps to give instruction in preparing meat, rice, soup, coffee, and tea. By 1863 an impressed Congress authorized the hiring of cooks to supervise the food preparation of every company mess hall detail. These units of one hundred men were the most convenient for instructing and serving. The Commission also recommended that each company also have its own fund for purchasing fresh fruits, vegetables, milk, butter, and condiments to supplement the usually plentiful rations.

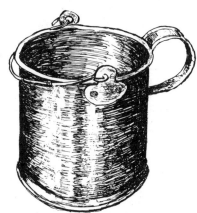

THE MESS CUP WAS LARGE ENOUGH TO USE AS A COOKING POT.

Under less control and more risk was the cooking in the field. Individual soldiers, tentmates, or up to a squad of twenty-five men could cook to their liking or pool their rations. But such catch-as-catch-can eating could be disasterous. The Commission found that after campaigning for three months of unsupervised cooking, 40 percent of a regiment's fighting strength would be lost through intestinal problems. While stories of maggoty hardtack, rancid salt pork, and salt beef jawbreakers may have filled the soldier's letters to home, his real complaints should have been the poorly prepared indigestibles that filled his stomach.

Yet individual cooking with the right know-how could be an answer to mealtime monotony. Take for example the disguising of salt pork as part of lobscouse ~ or especially that most popular meal in the army, baked beans. On bivouac, a flat stone was placed at the bottom of a dug baking hole and a fire built within it to burn for several hours. Water and a teaspoonful of soda were added to a quart of beans in a mess pot and boiled over the flames for twenty or thirty minutes. The water was poured off and replaced with just water and boiled until the beans were soft. A chunk of pork was placed in the middle and some salt and pepper added for seasoning. The coals were then scooped from the hole, the pot centered with a

UTENSILS USED BY JOHN SHURTLEFF, CO.F, 2ND MASSACHUSETTS CALVARY, UNTIL HIS DEATH IN A BALTIMORE MILITARY HOSPITAL, OCTOBER 30TH, 1864.

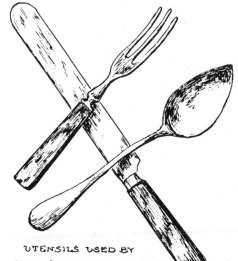

KNIFE AND SPOON COMBINATION WITH PATENT DATE, SEPTEMBER 17, 1861, FOR USE BY SOLDIERS WHO HAVE HAD ONE ARM AMPUTATED. GETTYSBURG NATIONAL MILITARY PARK

slab of wood or a preheated flat stone on top. Next the coals were banked around the pot, lengths of green saplings were cut long enough to span the hole, a piece of sacking or some old material laid over the saplings, and a mound of dirt was shoveled over the whole. If prepared the night of arrival at the campsite, some mighty fortunate soldiers would be having their Boston-style beans for breakfast the next morning.

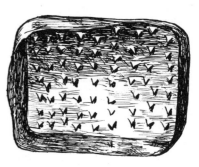

The Confederate army was a study of contrasts. The agricultural South converted many of its farms and cotton plantations into vast acreages of corn, wheat, rice, peas, and potatoes. With its slave labor to plant and harvest the crops, the early months of the war resembled an unending banquet of good things to eat. Yet by 1863 the Rebel army was limping along on half rations, grateful for any Union supplies that could be captured and whatever foraging that turned up in their line of march.

The reasons were several. By 1862 the Southern railroads were wearing out and the industrial North wasn't about to send along replacements. Within a year, backed-up stocks of produce lay moldering in depots and warehouses, all badly needed by the troops. Compounding the problem was an

SARDINE CAN MADE INTO A CORN
SHREDDER BY A CIVIL WAR SOLDIER.
GETTYSBURG NATIONAL MILITARY PARK.

inefficient Commissary Department that seemed to be constantly tripping over its own red tape. There were also less than patriotic farmers who held back on their harvests as prices rose and the Confederate currency nose-dived. Fighting hunger had become as much of a problem as fighting the Yankees.

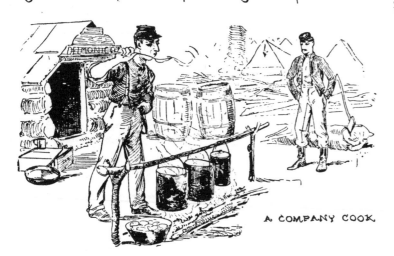

A COMPANY COOK.

PACKAGES FROM HOME

The morale boosters from the families back home were much appreciated—if they arrived as intended. Mary Livermore observed that Union "women rifled their storerooms and preserve closets of canned fruits and pots of jam and marmalade, which they packed with clothing and blankets, books and stationery and photographs. Baggage cars were soon flooded with fermenting sweetmeats and broken pots of jelly. Decaying fruits and vegetables, pastry and cake, badly canned meats and soups ruined clothing and papers." Fortunately the Sanitary Commission was able to sidestep the governmental tie-ups by receiving all such packages at their warehouses. There the goods and goodies would be repacked and sent directly to the soldiers, marked with the official Sanitation identification.

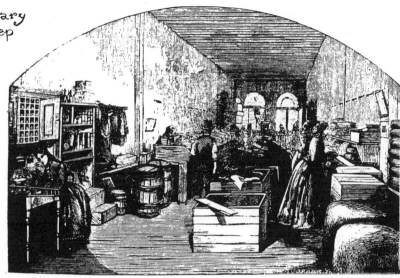

OFFICE OF A SOLDIERS' AID SOCIETY TO THE SANITARY COMMISSION

Unfortunately the Confederate troops had no Sanitation Commission to look out for their health and welfare. But when many of the packages had been lost or broken, a network of delivery was begun through Soldier Relief Societies, friends, relatives, travelers, and soldiers returning from furlough. Hand-delivered fresh vegetables, fried chicken, and sweets made up the bulk of the packages. And there were more modest requests such as Private George W. Athey's to send "alofe of lite bread and abig potatoe." Other wish lists included tomato catsup, pepper pickles, butter, apple butter, buckwheat bread, and sausages.

CAMP SUTLERS

The army sutler was a civilian shopkeeper specializing in a variety of foods, dry goods, and high prices. Usually every regiment, corps, or detachment had one such business stationed hard by the encampment in his hospital-style tent. Featured on display were the more recent foods to be encased in tin-canned meats, fruits, vegetables, and condensed milk.* Such exotic fare usually found its way to the officers' mess. More common sales might include sugar, molasses, and flour to the soldier who ran out of his rations, or a twist of tobacco for an after-dinner pipeful. Popular in Union camps were the relatively inexpensive molasses cookies and the rather skimpy pies. Sutlers did sell ardent spirits to 31 Union regiments, but the remaining 169 regiments had no such privilege.

As early as 1861 a newspaper attached to Joseph E. Johnston's Confederate command reported the sutler's profits to be several hundred percent. This did not sit kindly with Rebel soldiers and officers alike ~ particularly when such small luxuries as ginger cakes, half moon pies,

THE SUTLER'S TENT

and dried fruits skyrocketed in price. On more than one occasion, the encamped men became so enraged that they drove the rascally sutler out of camp and appropriated his offerings. It made more sense for the soldiers to purchase fresh produce from the local farmers, and in the event that any countryman overcharged,

*ALTHOUGH SALMON, LOBSTER, AND OYSTERS WERE FIRST CANNED IN 1819 AND THE VARIETY OF EDIBLES IN TIN CANS INCREASED WITHIN SIX YEARS, WIDE USAGE DIDN'T COME UNTIL AFTER THE WAR.

the military might give permission to seize any such edibles without payment.

CLOTHING

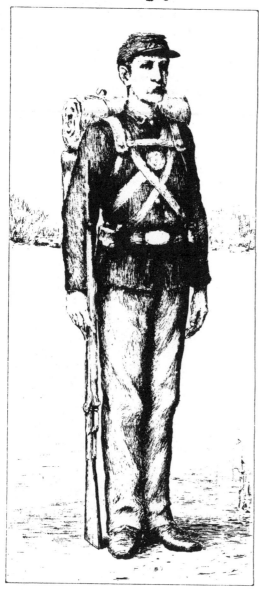

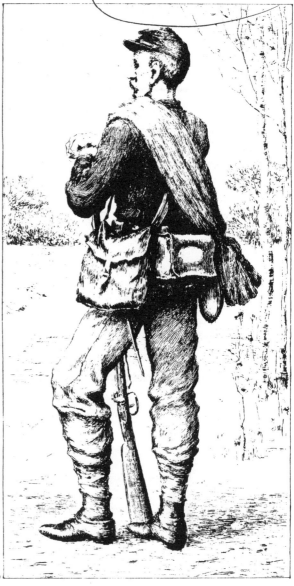

The newly mustered Union soldier received the same uniform and equipment as everyone else in line. He'd have his fatigue cap or occasionally a hat, a jacket~ otherwise known as a blouse that could serve as a dress coat~ an overcoat, one pair of shoes, one pair of pants, two flannel shirts, two flannel underdrawers, two pair of woolen socks, one woolen and one rubber blanket, a knapsack, haversack, canteen, and eating utensils. On the march he'd be burdened with a Minie or Sharps rifle, up to eighty rounds of ammunition, at least three day's rations, and half a shelter tent.

As warm weather approached, the line of march was often outlined by a litter of blankets and overcoats. Veterans had learned to bring along only the clothes on their backs and such necessities as the knapsack and haversack. Before charging the enemy, these carryalls would be put to one side

A SEASONED VETERAN ON CAMPAIGN

26

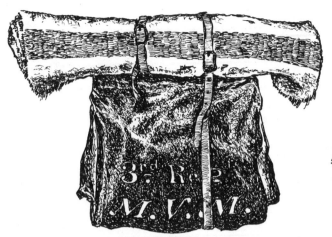

THE UNION KNAPSACK WAS THE SOLDIER'S HOME AWAY FROM HOME. IT COULD HOLD SIXTY ROUNDS OF AMMUNITION, A WOOLEN AND A RUBBER BLANKET, OVERCOAT, EXTRA SHIRT, DRAWERS, SOCKS, AND HALF A SHELTER TENT — ABOUT SIXTY POUNDS.

and recovered if all went well. Only if government-issue goods were lost in action would they be replaced. When the soldier's tour of duty had ended, the rifle, knapsack, haversack, and shelter tent would be turned in to the company's commanding officer.

An optimistic Confederate command listed clothing specifications that were similar to the Federal Army regulations. But gearing up for the manufacture of uniforms just couldn't compete with the North's industrial capabilities. Recruits might turn up in their flashy militia uniforms and would make first-rate targets compared to the cadet gray standard. Wearing captured Union uniforms was risky and could invite friendly fire, but not if the pants and jacket were dyed a butternut color. This yellowish-brown shade could be made locally of copperas and walnut hulls, and this unofficial Confederate color was so common that the Southern troops were known as "butternuts."

Six months after hostilities began, the Rebel troops were becoming a ragtag army. Most carried "housewives," otherwise known as sewing kits, to repair what they could — and often with a sense of humor. The Life of Johnny Reb made mention of a ranking system whereby "one hole in the seat of the breeches indicated a captain, two holes a lieutenant, and the seat of the pants all but out indicates that the individual is a private." Some letters home told of a "flag of truce" displayed on the backside of their pants. But any award for artistic patches in that same threadbare region might go to a large red flannel heart worn by one soldier, or perhaps to others with eagles, horses, cows, cannon, and even a cupid with a bow.

At least the Southern troops seemed to have plenty of socks, shirts, and underwear to combat exposure to the elements. The inflammation theory warned of improper dress risking pleurisy, quinsy throats, rheumatism, and a host of other illnesses from lowered bodily resistance. It was then the belief that flannel should be worn in all kinds of weather to encourage the pores of the skin to rid the body of "perspirable humors." It was

PACKED AND READY FOR THE MARCH

27

believed that sweating should not be inhibited by too little clothing, drinking excessive amounts of water, lying on a damp ground, or sitting in the wind.

Winter stockings were generally of wool, with fine lamb's wool being considered less likely to chafe the feet. Cotton or linen socks might be chosen for the warm months. Although machine-made stockings with seams were being manufactured in the North, they could not be turned out in the quantities needed by the Union troops. It was just as well, for the seam that ran the length of the stocking was irritating to the skin. The best answer, then, for both Northern and Southern troops, was the hand-knit wool stockings sent from the home front. Meanwhile the campaigning foot soldier who might raise a crop of foot sores on the road had best rub his feet with oil, fat, or a tallow candle as a preventive measure.

Of all the pieces of a soldier's uniform, shoes gave the wearer the greatest concern. According to the thinking of the times, shoes should have thick soles with an inner layer of cork or felt for protection against cold and dampness. All boots and shoes were fitted closely to the instep and were otherwise rather loose to prevent chafing. Ideally the shoes were broader and longer than the feet to prevent pressure and crowding of the toes—and, of course, to allow those "perspirable humors" to escape. And at the end of a hard march, The Military Handbook warned that nothing was more tempting ~ or dangerous ~ than plunging one's feet into cold water. It was the inflammatory theory at work again (see Sidelight 1 on footwear).

A FOOTSORE STRAGGLER

Before the first year of the Civil War was over, the Confederate soldier's most urgent clothing need was shoes. This was a marching army frequently on the attack, and the failing Southern Railroad system could offer little help. The Rebels' 1862 offensive into Maryland lost thousands of its soldiers along the way to worn-out footwear and the sorry state of their feet. Although the Confederate Congress had contracted with some 2,000 workers to hurry the badly needed shoes along, the problem was never really resolved. In desperation some army segments traded the commissary's meal-on-the-hoof rawhides for leather. The soldiers could then craft their own shoes or moccasins. Another possible after-battle source gave rise to the saying that "all a Yankee is worth is his shoes."

PATRIOTIC UNION WOMEN SUPPLIED 20,000 WHITE LINEN AND FLANNEL HAVELOCKS TO THE TROOPS FOR PROTECTION FROM STRONG SUNLIGHT. SUMMER'S HUMIDITY AND HEATED NECKS MADE DISCARDS OF THESE WELL INTENTIONED BUT USELESS GIFTS.

At the other end of the Civil War soldier rested his hat. There he displayed his specialty, perhaps a bugle for the infantry, two crossed cannons for the artillery, and the crossed sabers for the cavalry. The visor of the fatigue cap and the broad brim of the hat gave protection from the sun and rain. Coldness and dampness, those breeders of inflammation and its consequences, could be minimized. It was said that sunstroke could also be prevented by placing a silk handkerchief in the crown of the hat.

The importance of the hat gave rise to several well-meaning but ill-conceived head protectors. Early in the war, the New York Zouaves and their Southern Louisiana Zouave counterparts wore their distinctive tasseled Turkish fezes into battle. They were discarded when it was realized that they made outstanding targets.

Another idea that fell short of its mark was the havelock fuss. These neck-and-ear hat drapes might protect Union soldiers from the sun, thought Superintendent of Female Nurses Dorothea Dix, and she suggested to the Women's Central Association of Relief that 20,000 havelocks might be of great benefit to the military. Although without the blessing of the Sanitary Commission, the women made good on the request. Unfortunately the thick, coarse white linen and flannel covering collected the heat and was soon history.

The very practical Union army poncho was of unbleached muslin coated with vulcanized India rubber. The oblong was 71 inches long and 60 inches wide with a lengthwise centered opening for the head, and a neck lap 16 inches long and 3 inches wide. It doubled as a waterproof tent floor, allowing the soldier a dry night's sleep on the damp earth ~ another inflammation preventive.

It was with considerable pleasure that United States Sanitary Commission spokesman Olmsted reported to the secretary of war that "never probably, was so large an army as well supplied at a similar period of a great war."

BUTTON BOARD USED WHEN POLISHING UNIFORM BUTTONS

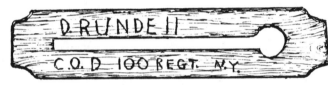

DRUNDELL

C.O.D 100 REGT. N.Y.

OWNED BY DANIEL DRUNDELL, CO. D., NEW YORK VOLUNTEER INFANTRY ~ GETTYSBURG NATIONAL MILITARY PARK

SHELTER

The wall tent, otherwise known as the hospital tent, had sidewalls that gave additional standing room. It dated from before the Colonial and Revolutionary Wars and had a proven track record. As a field hospital, it could shelter twenty patients. Two hospital tents could be joined at their ends, thereby doubling the capacity. Because of their size and bulk, they had to be transported by wagon during campaigns. A smaller size was used by general field and staff officers.

HOSPITAL TENT

All wall tents were topped with a fly. This oblong sheet of canvas provided an air space to keep the heat of the sun and the chill of the rain away from the tent top. The walls could be raised for airing. This all-season tent could be quite homey in the dead of winter if one end were blocked by a makeshift fireplace and given a heavy coating of clay. Scrounged stone and bricks could be mortared with local clay, becoming more hardened and permanent as the fireplace saw use.

Lacking noncombustibles for the chimney, pieces of split wood could be stacked in crosswise layers atop the fireplace and given a heavy coating of clay. A bit more risky was the substitution of pork or beef barrels for the upper reaches of the chimney. Occasionally one would catch fire, giving

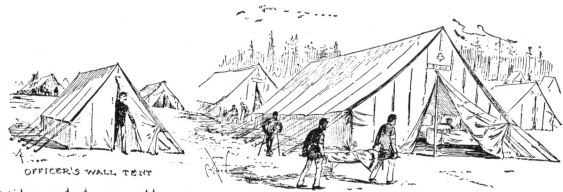

OFFICER'S WALL TENT

HOSPITAL WALL TENT

a bit of excitement to an otherwise ho-hum day at a Union or Confederate winter encampment.

The A or wedge tent was also common to both armies, although the Confederate quartermaster general was always playing catch-up to the tenting needs of the troops. It was a simple matter to pitch this single piece of canvas, but its height and length of 6 feet could cover only 7 square feet of ground space for all of its four occupants. The angled sides limited this space, and standing inside was a problem. If necessity called for the crowding in of five or six men for sleeping, they would have to fit together like a stack of spoons and turn over at the same time.

The unenthusiastic tenants were privates and noncommissioned officers, although a line officer might have such a tent to himself when on a march. The Sanitary Commission had hard words to say about the inability to raise the sides for airing and cleaning.

A OR WEDGE TENTS

Longer-term winter encampments allowed for a more comfortable A-tent lifestyle. The first winter of 1861 gave Northern and Southern troops time enough to raise a log or split-log wall frame ~ really a log-notched cabin with a canvas roof. Digging out a foot or two of floor sod within the framework produced a shelter that gave more warmth and headroom. At one end would be the fireplace and its chimney, a snug arrangement to await the coming of spring. This bulky yardage of canvas was more suited for semipermanent living than for transporting on the campaign trail. The Union army came up with a better idea: the single-shelter tent.

The single shelter, or half shelter, was better known as a dog or pup tent ~ and there wasn't much more room than that to spare. It was born of experience late in 1861, for it was light enough for every Union foot soldier to carry with ease while freeing the wagons to carry more food and ammunition.

DIVERSION AT A LOG-WALLED TENT ENCAMPMENT

Actually it was only half a tent~ an oblong of canvas about 5 feet 2 inches long by 4 feet 8 inches wide. Three of its edges had a row of buttons and buttonholes plus loops at the ends of the fourth edge for tent pegs. Two soldiers would buddy up and button up to join their halves. There was no need to level the woods for ridgepoles and their tent pole supports. Instead two rifles with fixed bayonets, thrust into the ground, could then be connected with rope at their trigger guards for a quick and efficient two-man shelter.

In 1864 the Union Quartermaster General's office enlarged the pup tent halves to 5 feet 6 inches in length by 5 feet 5 inches. The cotton duck fabric held nine galvanized metal buttons along its upper edge and seven running down each short side. In addition there would be twenty-three matching buttonholes to accept another half shelter. Loops of a six-thread manila rope were sewn to the corners and center of the lower edge. A ridge rope 6 feet 10 inches in length was also provided in the new do-it-yourself pup tent. In a winter encampment many dog tent halves could be joined to make a gabled roof over log or half-log sidings.

HALF-SHELTER TENT

CONFEDERATE SOLDIER JOHN ZIELER'S FIREWOOD AXE.

GOVERNMENT ISSUE MATCHES GETTYSBURG NATIONAL PARK

CLEANLINESS

The personal hygiene among Union troops received no passing grades in Olmsted's December 1861 report. The Sanitary Commission's inspectors found that the volunteer regimental officers were paying little if any attention to their troops' general health. Private D. L. Day of the 25th Massachusetts Volunteer Infantry put his Yankee ingenuity to work when he wrote about that time:

"I have been looking through the camp around here and am astonished at the amount of offal and swill that is buried up and lost instead of being turned into valuable account. An enterprising farmer could collect from these camps manure and swill to the value of $100 a day, costing nothing but simply carting it off, thus enriching his land and fattening hundreds of hogs and cattle; but this lack of energy and enterprise prevents these people from turning anything to account. They content themselves with sitting down and finding fault with the government and their more enterprising neighbors of the north."

The Confederate top brass were no less concerned about the lack of Rebel personal and camp cleanliness. General Robert E. Lee wrote in 1861 that "our poor sick I know suffer much, but they bring it on themselves by not doing what they are told. They are worse than children."

The Union's daily routine rules in "The Military Handbook & Soldiers Manual" of June 1861 were clear enough.

"Ordinarily the cleaning will be on Saturdays. The chiefs of the squads will cause bedding to be overhauled; floors dry rubbed; tables and benches scoured; arms cleaned; accouterments whitened and polished, and everything put in order.

"Where conveniences for bathing are to be had, the men should bathe once a week. The feet to be washed at least twice a week. The hair kept short, and the beard neatly trimmed.

"Non-commissioned officers, in command of squads, will be held immediately responsible that their men observe what is prescribed above; that they wash their hands and faces daily; that they brush and comb their heads."

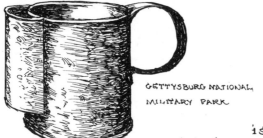

THE SHAVING BRUSH WAS USED BY SGT. EMANUEL BRALLIES, CO. D, 110TH PENNSYLVANIA VOLUNTEER INFANTRY. THE SHAVING CUP BELONGED TO ISAAC HARLOW, CO. A, 11TH NEW JERSEY VOLUNTEER INFANTRY.

GETTYSBURG NATIONAL MILITARY PARK

And on this subject, "The Military Handbook & Soldiers Manual notes "that excellent authority 'Hall's Journal of Health' advice to the Yankee soldiers. 'Let the whole beard grow, but no longer than three inches. This strengthens and thickens its growth, and makes a more perfect protection for the lungs against dust and of the throat against winds and colds in winter, while in the summer a greater perspiration of the skin is induced, with an increase in evaporation; hence greater coolness of the parts on the outside, while the throat is less feverish, thirsty and dry.'" The good doctor didn't say if all this facial fur could strain out such external stimuli as poisonous air ~ marsh fever or malaria ~ causing acute inflammation.

Dr. Hall offered other advice to the troops that seems ahead of his time. "Whenever it is possible, do, by all means, when you have to use water for cooking or drinking from ponds or sluggish streams, boil it well, and when cool, shake it or stir it, so that the oxygen of the air shall get into it, which greatly improves it for drinking. This boiling arrests the process of fermentation which arises from the presence of organic and inorganic impurities [the as yet undiscovered bacteria] this tending to prevent cholera and all bowel diseases."

Hall went on to say, "If there is no time for boiling, at least strain through a cloth, even if you have to use a shirt or trouser-leg." It was a rule of thumb that water was wholesome enough for drinking when the water appeared clear and had no unpleasant smell. Some soldiers carried small filtering devices to place in murky water. "Pure water" was absorbed into the porous mini-canteen and then sipped through its mouthpiece ~ along, of course, with any microorganisms present.

POCKET MIRROR USED BY PHILIP LEIDY, M.D. CIVIL WAR MUSEUM PHILADELPHIA, PENNSYLVANIA

When thousands of volunteers were crammed into a campsite, the sick list increased dramatically. While Surgeon General Finley seemed powerless to start corrective measures, the Sanitary Commission made better camp health their business: campsites should be elevated and well away from swampy low-lying areas that might give off "infectious currents." Tents must be well

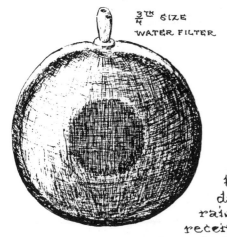

3TH SIZE
WATER FILTER

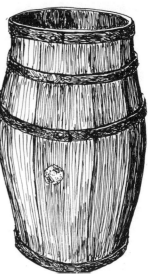

"THIS KEG WAS USED TO CARRY FRESH WATER TO THE WOUNDED AFTER THE ANTIETAM BATTLE, 1862."
GETTYSBURG NATIONAL PARK

distanced from their nearest neighbors, and the space between not used as the local dump. Privies ~ basically a board raised over a trench ~ should receive a daily covering of dirt. The Commission made it clear that both officers and men must have a better understanding of such health measures ~ and provide camp police to enforce them. As early as September 1861, Olmsted could report improvement to Washington, and "a small sick list meant higher spirits and morale."

CHANGING THE OLD GUARD

As 1861 drew to a close, the United States Sanitary Commission stepped up its campaign against the "ossified and useless" Surgeon General Finley. For too long he had been bogged down in a mire of inactivity and inefficiency. It was long past time for a change when the Commission presented Congress with a Medical Department reorganization bill ~ and it included a new surgeon general. Congress agreed, Finley was history, and the Commission's nominee, Dr. William A. Hammond, was approved by Washington April 25, 1862. Hammond was thirty-four years old ~ young indeed when compared with his ancient predecessors.

He was a man to look up to ~ above and beyond his 6-foot-2-inch frame, which carried 240 pounds of weight. He distinguished himself as an army assistant surgeon in the Indian campaigns by writing a number of papers and books on scurvy, hygiene, physiology, and health of the western Indians. He

SURGEON GENERAL WILLIAM HAMMOND

spent an extended leave in Europe studying in the best of their military hospitals. His reputation earned him a professorship of anatomy and physiology at the University of Maryland in 1859. At the outbreak of the Civil War, Hammond re-enlisted in the United States Army. He caught the notice of General George McClellan, who in turn suggested his name to the Commission as a well-qualified candidate for the surgeon general's post.

The new surgeon general came to his office primed with many reforms. A sampling included designing better records for the sick and wounded, establishing an army medical school, placing all ambulances, medical supplies, and hospital construction under the control of the surgeon general, establishing a permanent general hospital in Washington, and raising the rank and pay of army surgeons. But his first order of business was the safe and prompt removal of battlefield wounded to efficient field hospitals. A permanent ambulance and hospital corps staffed by trained medical department personnel were also musts.

"M.S." STANDS FOR MEDICAL STAFF AND WAS THE EARLIEST MEDICAL OFFICER INSIGNIA. THE EMBROIDERED SILVER INITIALS, SURROUNDED BY A GOLD WREATH, WERE WORN ON THE EPAULETTES.

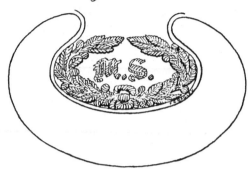

THE EMBLEM WAS WORN PRIOR TO THE 1845-47 MEXICAN WAR UNTIL 1872. THE INITIALS WERE CHANGED TO "M.D." AND WORN ON THE COLLAR UNTIL 1890.

THE AMBULANCE CORPS

Although ambulances played no part in the Mexican and the Indian Wars that followed, rumblings of secession gave life (unfortunately, the only signs of life in the United States Army Medical Bureau) to two prototypes in 1859. One was a four-wheeled wagon disguised as an ambulance by a rigging of canvas sides, with room enough

THE LARREY "FLYING AMBULANCE," 1797

for four patients in relative comfort; the second design, the "Coolidge" and the "Finley" two-wheeled ambulance models, could make no such claim.

The two wheelers were probably patterned after the French two-wheeled ambulances of 1797.

The two-wheelers were thought to be the best possible transportation for any dangerously ill or wounded soldier but trial and many errors found that the passengers between the two wheels rocked about like a child's see-saw. The Army of the Potomac had been allotted five of these "dandleboards"— much to its regret. In just three months of use, half of their number had mercifully broken down because of their light and basically weak construction.

THE PRE-WAR "COOLIDGE" AMBULANCE WAGON

There was a French ambulance of sorts that might be mentioned in passing. The new "cacolet" was simplicity itself: it could carry two wounded soldiers

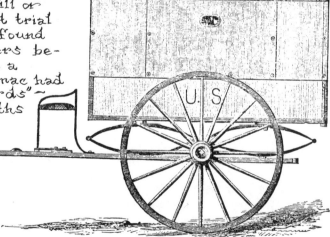

THE FINLEY ONE HORSE AMBULANCE WAGON

on the sides of a horse over any irregular terrain. Unfortunately, the patients were unable to lie down, because the motion of the horse gave an oppressive dizziness. This, plus its bulky 140-pound frame and the lack of protection from snow and rain proved the idea unworkable.

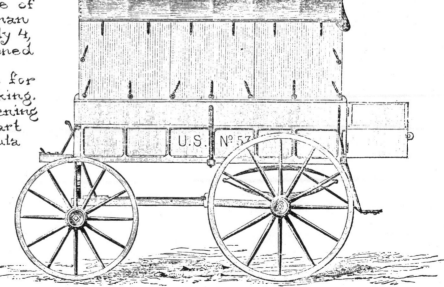

BRITISH CRIMEAN CACOLET

From the very beginning of the conflict, the Confederacy was ambulance poor. Wear and tear further reduced the number of ambulances available. The rescue problems of battlefield wounded were considerably less, however, than those during the first two years of the war. The Rebels' winning streak left each battlefield in their possession with time enough to remove the wounded by stretcher, horse litter, and pack mule to any nearby buildings that could serve as field hospitals. A more leisurely train ride to the various general hospitals would follow~ at least until the fortunes of the Federal forces improved.

Union ambulance efforts were headed in the right direction by February 1862. It was then that General Grant was moving his regiments by steamer transports down the Tennessee River for an offensive into Alabama. His medical director, Dr. John Brinton, reported that "all the ambulances were collected together for the formation of ambulance trains. Each of these trains was placed under the charge of a non-commissioned officer, whose business it was to see that a continuous line of wagons should ply between the scene of conflict and the general hospital. As a result, the majority of the wounded on the field were transported to points where every surgical attention could be rendered."

The next step~and a giant step it was~came from newly appointed Surgeon General Hammond. For the troubled Army of the Potomac, he nominated Surgeon Jonathan Letterman~the right man for the job.

The Peninsular Campaign drive had been hobbled by thousands of sick and wounded, a lack of medicine, and an inability to reach the battlefield wounded for up to a full week before rescue or death would carry them away (see Sidelight 2). It was with a real sense of urgency that Dr. Letterman reported for duty on July 4, 1862, to join a disheartened medical staff.

He was just in time for another crisis in the making. General Lee was threatening Washington, the very heart of the Union. The Peninsula Campaign was aborted. Troops hurrying to the defense of the capital were roundly defeated in a second Bull Run battle, and the successful Confederate troops were massing to cross the Potomac River near Antietam, Maryland, on August 2, 1862.

A PRE-CIVIL WAR FOUR-WHEELER, THE ROSECRANS AMBULANCE

In the desperate fighting that followed, Letterman's Ambulance Corps was able to remove each of the 10,000 wounded from the battlefield and to give treatment under adequate shelters within twenty-four hours. Many a wounded Union soldier must have become a believer in miracles that day

In just a month and a half, with the advice and experience of Surgeon General Hammond, Letterman had transformed the ambulance service by removing all individual regimental control. Instead, each army corps with two or more divisions would now have its own ambulance corps commanded by a captain. He would see that all men under him would follow the corps regulations, right down to such details as the front man carrying a stretcher stepping off with his left foot and the rear man with his right. Each ambulance division was led by a first lieutenant, each brigade by a second lieutenant, and each regiment by a sergeant. All of the officers were line

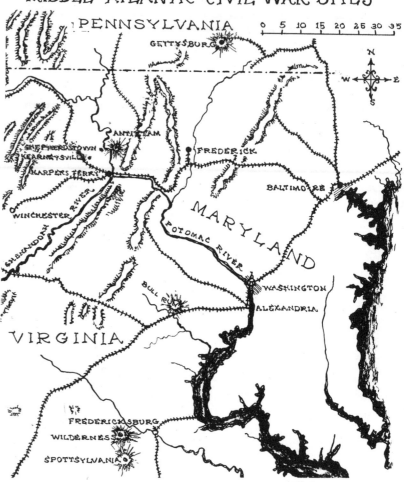

MIDDLE ATLANTIC CIVIL WAR SITES

officers, experienced leaders, and supervisors with specific duties in the heat of battle. The overall direction and control was in the capable hands of Letterman (see Sidelight 3).

Other officers were responsible for the upkeep of Letterman's new light, larger, and more comfortable soft-spring ambulances as well as the horses and their harnesses. They would see that a supply box under the driver's seat, under lock and key, held six two-pound cans of beef pork, three different sizes of camp kettles, six tin plates, six tin tumblers, six tablespoons, one lantern and candle, one leather bucket, and three bedsacks. Just before the fighting began, ten pounds of hard bread would be added to the box.

Each division would now keep its ambulances together as a train without any regimental control. On occasion the division trains might be combined to form a large corps train. As a rule of thumb, the number of ambulances in any train was about 1 for every 150 soldiers. Such were the essentials of Letterman's ambulance

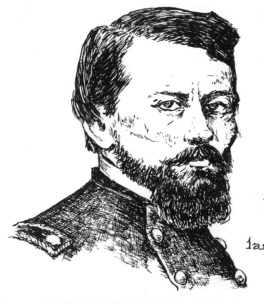

ARMY OF THE POTOMAC MEDICAL DIRECTOR JONATHAN LETTERMAN

corps. So successful were they, in fact, that the newly organized ambulance corps would become the blueprint for the entire United States Army.

There were other refinements. Each corps had its own reserve medicine wagon and every brigade an army wagon filled with the essential medicines, instruments dressings, bedding, basins, spoons, tumblers and similar hospital supplies ~ AND up-to-date reference books that previous surgeon generals thought a waste of money. The wounded Union soldier then, could count on a prompt rescue by the train of ambulances and a ride to the ambulance depot to the rear of the fighting. An assistant surgeon and his trained staff stood ready to give emergency first aid, stop any hemorrhaging, bandage the wounds, splint the fractures, give pain suppressants, and treat the shock.

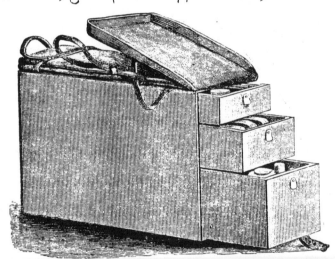

THE 1859 TRIPLER AMBULANCE COULD CARRY FOUR PRONE AND SIX SEATED SOLDIERS, BUT PROVED TOO HEAVY AND CUMBERSOME. ITS NAMESAKE DR. CHARLES S. TRIPLER WAS REPLACED BY LETTERMAN AS MEDICAL DIRECTOR, ARMY OF THE POTOMAC.

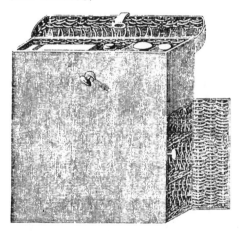

EACH UNION REGIMENTAL SURGEON WAS ISSUED A HOSPITAL KNAPSACK OF WICKERWORK COVERED WITH AN ENAMELED CLOTH DURING THE FIRST YEAR OF THE WAR.

THE REGULATION HOSPITAL KNAPSACK OF 1862 FOLLOWED BUT PROVED TO BE TOO HEAVY AND CUMBERSOME.

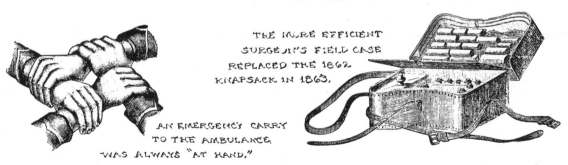

THE MORE EFFICIENT SURGEON'S FIELD CASE REPLACED THE 1862 KNAPSACK IN 1863.

AN EMERGENCY CARRY TO THE AMBULANCE WAS ALWAYS "AT HAND."

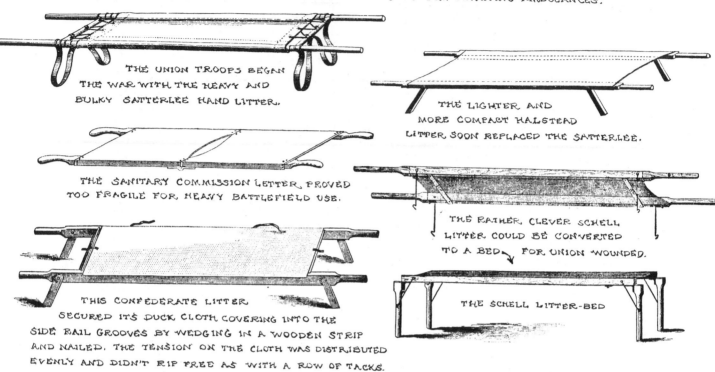

HAND LITTERS WERE A GOOD DEAL MORE EFFICIENT THAN HAND-CLASPED SEATS WHEN CARRYING THE WOUNDED OFF THE BATTLEFIELD TO TO THE AWAITING AMBULANCES.

THE UNION TROOPS BEGAN THE WAR WITH THE HEAVY AND BULKY SATTERLEE HAND LITTER.

THE LIGHTER AND MORE COMPACT HALSTEAD LITTER SOON REPLACED THE SATTERLEE.

THE SANITARY COMMISSION LITTER PROVED TOO FRAGILE FOR HEAVY BATTLEFIELD USE.

THE RATHER CLEVER SCHELL LITTER COULD BE CONVERTED TO A BED FOR UNION WOUNDED.

THIS CONFEDERATE LITTER SECURED ITS DUCK CLOTH COVERING INTO THE SIDE RAIL GROOVES BY WEDGING IN A WOODEN STRIP AND NAILED. THE TENSION ON THE CLOTH WAS DISTRIBUTED EVENLY AND DIDN'T RIP FREE AS WITH A ROW OF TACKS.

THE SCHELL LITTER-BED

The Battle of Antietam, September 17-18, 1862, became a proving ground for Letterman's ambulance plan and an indictment against the previous uncoordinated and often haphazard retrieval and care of its casualties. The Confederate Army, still under those timeworn regulations that worked well enough in a small peacetime yesterday, soon found itself in desperate straits (see Sidelight 3). Southerner Mary Bedenger Mitchell described the evacuation of the rebel wounded at nearby Shepherdstown:

"Monday afternoon we suddenly found the wounded in our streets, what seemed to be an endless line of wagons discharging their piteous burdens. There were no preparations, no accommodations, not even a courier in advance to announce their arrival. The men could not be left in the streets; men ran for keys and unlocked unused buildings. Hay was brought and covered with blankets; on these improvised beds the sufferers were placed, and the next question was how to dress their wounds. No surgeons were to be seen. A few men detailed as nurses had come but they were incompetent. Our women set heartily to work; washed, bandaged, bathed and did what they could without knowledge or experience. Every housekeeper ransacked her stores for material for bandages. The doctors came by and by; some rough surgery was done, mostly amputating. [These surgeons did not impress Mrs. Mitchell favorably.]

"This was Monday, the day after the battle of South Mountain. Next day fresh wounded poured in, and they worked all day. This day would have brought despair for food, but an apology for the commissary arrived; also some additional doctors, most of whom might as well have stayed away.

"On Wednesday the battle began again, this time so near that the roar of artillery and the rattle of musket fire was heard from dawn to dark. The wounded before had been but a prelude. Now they came in thousands, absolutely deluging the little country village. In the streets was noise, confusion, dust, throngs of stragglers, horsemen, wagons blocking each other; and a continual din of shouting, swearing, and rumbling, in the midst of which men were dying, fresh wounded arriving, surgeons amputating and women going in and out with bandages, lint, medicines, and food. The wounded continued to arrive until the town was quite unable to hold all the disabled and suffering; they filled every building and overflowed into the country around. Those able to travel were sent on to Winchester and other towns, but their removal seemed to make no appreciable difference.

"On Thursday night we heard more than the usual sounds, and in the morning we found the Confederates in full retreat. General Lee crossed the Potomac under cover of darkness and moved toward Kearneysville. General McClellan followed to the river and began shelling the retreating army, and consequently the town. What before was confusion grew infinitely worse. The roads were thronged, the streets blocked, and the wounded started off in crowds. In vain we implored them to stay. They replied that the Yankees were crossing, the town was to be burned, that we could not be made prisoners but they could, that anyhow they were going ~ and go they did. Men with cloths about their heads went hatless in the sun; men with injured feet limped shoeless on the stony road; men in ambulances, wagons, carts, wheelbarrows, on stretchers, or supported on the shoulder of some comrade ~ all who could crawl went, and almost to certain death. They could not go far, they dropped off in the country houses; but their wounds had become inflamed; erysiplas or gangrine followed and long rows of nameless graves bear witness to the results."

Mary Mitchell also pointed up some of the regimental field hospital problems: isolation from the others, massive numbers of casualties, little skilled help and medicines, and lack of mobility if the enemy should advance on their position.

THE VERSATILE ROLLER BANDAGE WAS APPLIED MORE TIGHTLY AT ITS MOST DISTANT POINT AND GRADUALLY LOOSENED AS THE BANDAGE ASCENDED. WHEN THE LIMB INCREASED IN SIZE, THE BANDAGE WAS TURNED ON ITSELF TO LIE SMOOTHLY.

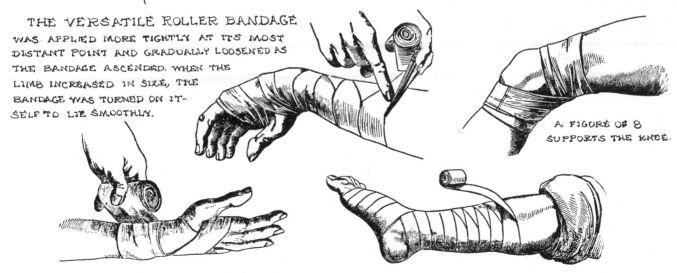

A FIGURE OF 8 SUPPORTS THE KNEE.

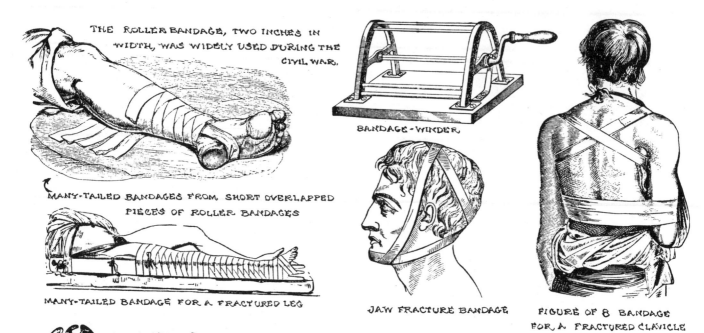

THE ROLLER BANDAGE, TWO INCHES IN WIDTH, WAS WIDELY USED DURING THE CIVIL WAR.

BANDAGE-WINDER

MANY-TAILED BANDAGES FROM SHORT OVERLAPPED PIECES OF ROLLER BANDAGES

MANY-TAILED BANDAGE FOR A FRACTURED LEG

JAW FRACTURE BANDAGE

FIGURE OF 8 BANDAGE FOR A FRACTURED CLAVICLE

A NEW DIVISIONAL FIELD HOSPITAL PLAN

In the days gone by, the regimental field hospital would have been the next stop for the ambulance and its wounded cargo. Jonathan Letterman's circular letter of October 30, 1862, told of more changes coming to the Army of the Potomac. As its medical director, he announced that the new plan would mean "that the wounded may receive the most prompt and efficient attention during and after an engagement by the most skillful and responsible Surgeons at the earliest moment."

The plan was this: all regimental field hospitals would be consolidated into divisional field hospitals during battle. This meant that three regiments would make up each division of about fifteen thousand or more men (see Sidelight 3). Those who fell in battle would continue on their ride from the ambulance depot emergency care to each division field hospital site previously selected by the corps medical director.

In this protected site the divisional ambulances would be standing ready

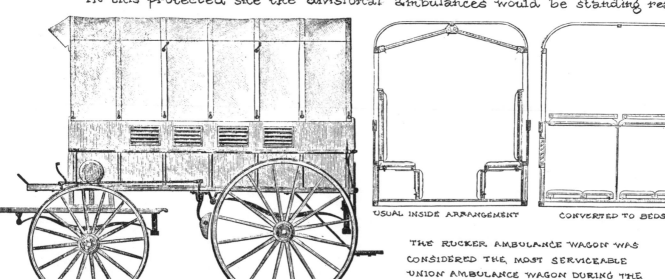

USUAL INSIDE ARRANGEMENT

CONVERTED TO BEDS

THE RUCKER AMBULANCE WAGON WAS CONSIDERED THE MOST SERVICEABLE UNION AMBULANCE WAGON DURING THE LATTER PART OF THE WAR.

and under the direction of an assistant surgeon. As detailed by the divisional surgeon-in-chief, he would see that their hospital wagon was well stocked with arrowroot, tea, coffee, and like refreshments. He would ready a shelter for the incoming wounded with hospital tents and straw, blankets, water, and similar articles of comfort. Any hospital cooks, stewards, and nurses that might be needed would be under his command.

The divisional surgeon-in-chief, under the direction of the corps medical director, also selected three medical officers to be responsible for all major operations. Their selection from the regiments would be made with great care and determined without regard to rank or seniority. They would be of prudent judgment and known for their concern for the well-being of their patients. Each of the three surgeons would have an assistant surgeon under his direction. One of these assistants would administer the anesthetic, and each operating surgeon would be supplied with "an excellent table" from the hospital wagon— no more jury-rigged operating tables from old doors or the backs of wagons (see Sidelight 4 for instruments carried in the medicine wagons).

The third assistant surgeon kept a record of every patient brought to the division field hospital. In the past the family and friends made a postbattle search of the battlefield or the regimental field hospital with little hope that any information or direction could be given by the army. Now a complete record of every case would include the name, rank, company and regiment, the injury described, and the treatment and results detailed. The third assistant surgeon would ensure that there was a proper interment of the dead, including a grave "headboard" bearing the name, rank, company, and regiment of the soldier.

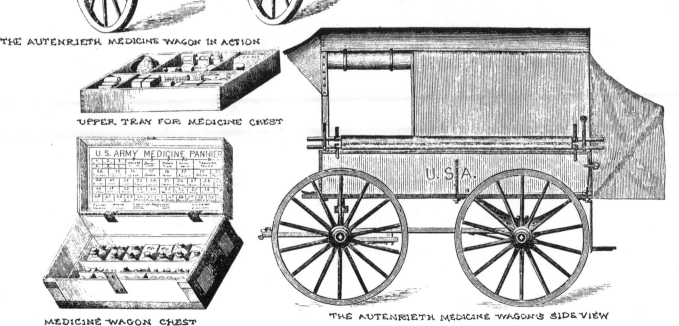

THE AUTENRIETH MEDICINE WAGON IN ACTION

UPPER TRAY FOR MEDICINE CHEST

U.S. ARMY MEDICINE PANNIER

MEDICINE WAGON CHEST

THE AUTENRIETH MEDICINE WAGON'S SIDE VIEW

Every brigade surgeon-in-chief would issue supplies as needed to re-stock each regimental medicine chest and the hospital knapsack used by a regimental first-aid officer (see Sidelight 5). He would be stationed a safe distance behind his regiment to give initial help to the battlefield wounded. Many with less severe wounds could reach this station under their own power and not have need of the ambulance corps. All other unassigned medical officers in the division would act as general assistants and dressers in the division field hospital.

Letterman's innovative field hospital changes were put to the test in the Fredericksburg campaign. On December 13, 1862, Major General Burnside ordered an ill-conceived attack across the Rappahannock River against well-entrenched Confederate forces. In the disaster that followed, his lack of perception accounted for a needless 1,200 dead and 9,000 wounded Union soldiers. But for the first time, those still among the living could agree with the report submitted by Medical Director J. T. Heard, U.S. Volunteers. He said, "In no previous battle witnessed by me were the wounded so promptly and well cared for throughout the army as at Fredericksburg. This was due to the uniformity of action. Every surgeon, hospital steward, nurse, cook, and attendant was assigned his position and knew it."

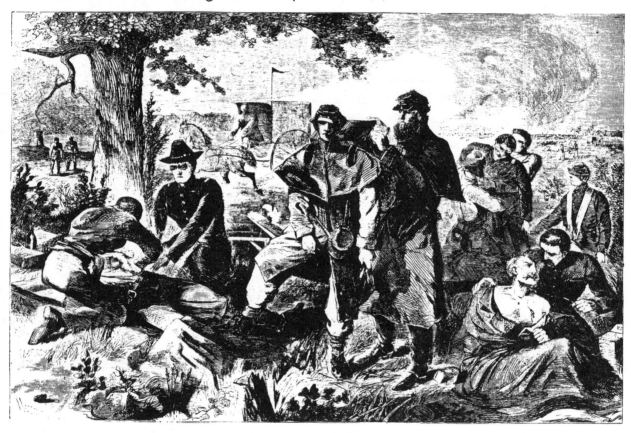

SURGEON AT WORK DURING AN ENGAGEMENT (WINSLOW HOMER)

WHILE HOMER WAS A STAFF ARTIST FOR "HARPER'S WEEKLY" HE SKETCHED THIS CIVIL WAR SCENE FROM LIFE AND SENT IT NORTHWARD TO BE ENGRAVED ON WOOD. IT WAS PUBLISHED IN THAT WEEKLY IN NEW YORK, 1862.

FIELD HOSPITAL ANESTHESIA

Being assigned to the field hospital was hardly an honor, for all who qualified might well undergo major surgery. The consolation prize was chloroform,* the anesthetic of choice for capital operations in both Union and Rebel armies. Whatever the fate of a wounded limb, a painfree unconsciousness could be counted upon during the cutting.

The 1863 <u>Manual of Military Surgery</u> <u>Prepared for the Use of the Confederate States Army</u> gave all the practicalities of administering anesthetics. Briefly, it stated that chloroform should be given in the fresh air with the patient's head on a pillow and the body remaining horizontal throughout the inhalation. The clothing should be loosened about the neck, chest, and abdomen so that breathing is not restricted. Only a light but nutritious meal should be given earlier, or the state of unconsciousness during the second stage of the anesthetic might bring on vomiting.

Before the chloroform was to be given, it was the "universal practice" in the Confederate Army to first give brandy (the Union surgeons generally used alcoholic stimuli only on physically depressed patients because they felt it could slow down the induction of anesthesia in a healthy patient). Sometimes a few drops of laudanum were helpful, and the surgeon was always to reassure the patient that any feeling of suffocation would soon disappear.

The Confederate manual went on to say that "all special instruments of inhalation have been discarded, and a towel or napkin, folded into a cone, by having its corners turned down, is now almost universally employed for the purpose. The chloroform, about a drachm [or $\frac{1}{8}$ ounce] is poured into this cone, and is held over the patient's mouth and nostrils which should previously have been anointed." By holding the cone a half inch from the patient's face, facial blistering was prevented and an adequate amount of air inhaled.

The first stage of chloroform was one of excitement ~ "muttering, wild eyed, the cries, the exaulted imagination" followed by "violent struggles, attempts to rise, and rigid contraction." Here if the spasm extended to the larynx, there would be danger of the breathing being obstructed. Removing the cone temporarily should give enough fresh air. While giving the anesthetic, the anesthetist should pay the "strictest attention to the condition of the respiration, pulse, and countenance."

The second stage was one of unconsciousness, insensibility, and relaxation of the voluntary muscles. The patient could not be aroused and the eyelids no

---

* DR. SAMUEL GUTHRIE OF SACKETS HARBOR, NEW YORK, WAS THE FIRST TO DISTILL CHLORIDE OF LIME WITH ALCOHOL IN A COPPER STILL IN 1831. HE CALLED IT CHLORIC ETHER SOON TO BE NAMED "CHLOROFORM."

longer contracted when touched. The pulse would be slow and weak and respiration shallow and feeble. If a respiratory obstruction were to occur in the second stage, the problem would be muscle relaxation with the epiglottis falling over the glottis. Danger signs would include an ashen skin, an overly distended neck, dilatation of the pupils, heavy snoring, and a cool skin. Death would be close at hand. Inhalation must be stopped immediately and the tongue seized and drawn out forcibly to clear the obstructed glottis. Plenty of fresh cold air must be given, as well as cold water on the face and chest, a stimulating enema, "and if to be had at once, electricity is applied."

Experience seemed to be the best and often the only teacher when using the recently discovered chloroform. This great boon to surgery was nonflammable, bland smelling, and rapid acting — but had to be used with caution. A prompt and efficient dose with enough fresh air would be administered at the outset of the operation. Enough would be used to last through the most difficult part of the surgery, then discontinued for a smoother recovery. As for those cases with injuries unattended well beyond the twenty-four-hour primary operative period and in an exhausted state, they should receive no anesthetic at all.

A PERIOD
MAGNETO ELECTRIC MACHINE

Ether had its own pluses and minuses. It was slow acting, had a disagreeable smell that patients resisted, and increased the cough reflex — all qualities that made few friends in the hard-pressed field hospitals. Yet it was frequently used in the Federal general hospitals where surgery was less pressing. It had none of chloroform's tendency to cause vomiting, prostration, and increased excitement.

The Union Army had records of but four deaths from ether during the entire Civil War period, while chloroform was involved in 5.4 deaths for every thousand soldiers who received it. Perhaps the experiences of Dr. William Morton, the dentist who proved ether's worth to the world back in 1846, had some influence on this remarkable record. He had given courses in anesthesia to the Union surgeons at the request of General Grant.

THE ETHER DRIP BOTTLE WAS AVAILABLE BUT LITTLE USED.

The Confederate anesthetic supply was a sometimes thing. The Secessionists, faced with a limited ability to manufacture pharmaceuticals plus an effective Yankee blockade on imports, had to use chloroform and ether sparingly. This was especially so because more of the volatile liquid evaporated into the air than into the patient when a handkerchief nose cone was used.

Confederate surgeon Julian John Chisolm came up with an ingenious device: a flattened cylinder that was 2½ inches long and 1 inch wide at its broadest diameter. Two nose tubes could be raised for use or pushed inside the inhaler for carrying in one's pocket. To load, chloroform was dripped into a per-

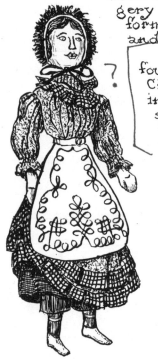

THIS 1851 RAG DOLL WAS SIMILAR TO THOSE USED TO SMUGGLE ETHER THROUGH UNION LINES FOR REBEL USE.

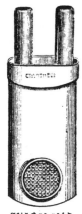

forated disc and onto an interior sponge or cloth. The patient would inhale chloroform through the nose tubes as it mixed with air drawn in through the perforated disc. Best of all, only an eighth of an ounce of the anesthetic was needed as opposed to the one or two ounces used with the handkerchief cone.

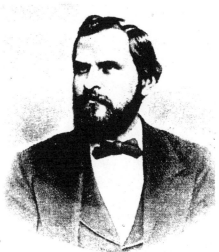

Anesthetics were used well over 80,000 times in the conflict by Union surgeons. Despite a meager supply, the Confederate usage might have come close to that figure. Gone were the days of "biting the bullet," for midcentury medicine had made real progress in this new surgical pain relief. As for surgery itself, the Civil War brought no major advances other than the technical skills learned from the overwhelming demands at the field hospitals.

CHISOLM'S INHALER

JULIAN J. CHISOLM, M.D.

FIELD HOSPITAL SURGERY

All battlefield wounds (see Sidelight 6) welcomed an assortment of rapidly multiplying bacteria well before the patient reached the field hospital. Since surgeons had no knowledge of the germ theory, sterile operating conditions would have made no sense. A slosh of water was good enough to clear a bloody operating table, the same old sponges and rinse water would wash the wound, and the contaminated hands and instruments would add more germs to a site that needed no further insult. If all went well, "laudable" pus would be evidence of normal healing, provided the body could rally to its own defense to fight the unseen invaders (see Sidelight 7).

PROJECTILE WOUNDS

Ninety-four percent of all wounds suffered in the Civil War were from bullets. To the regret of those soldiers who got in the way of one, the less damaging spherical ball of past American wars had largely been replaced by the Minie bullet. French army Captain Claude Etienne Minie did the medical profession no favor when he invented the conical soft-lead rifle bullet. Its hollow base expanded when it was fired to fit into the spiral grooves of the bore. Like a present-day football pass, the bullet rotated on its longitudinal axis in a straight course. Its conical point had less resistance to the air, greatly increasing its velocity. The Civil War soldier now had in his hands a rifle that was deadly for a distant target.

The field hospital surgeon could tell a good

ROUND MUSKET BALL

BUCK & BALL

COLT'S ARMY PISTOL BULLET

SPRINGFIELD RIFLE BULLET

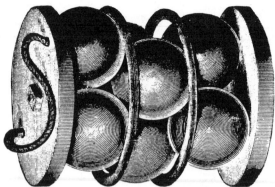

EVERY PIECE OF THE CANNON GRAPESHOT
CLUSTER BECAME A DEADLY PROJECTILE.

deal by examining the wound itself. An entrance hole without any exit could mean only that the bullet remained within the body. Before removing the soldier's uniform, he would check whatever lay over the wound: clothing, belt buckle, buttons, and the like. Fragments of clothing or metal would probably be carried along or perhaps the bullet had been deflected to make a less obvious pathway. The surgeon would use his finger to probe the wound, determine its direction, and to check for foreign bodies along the route.

CIVIL WAR BULLET PROBES AND FORCEPS

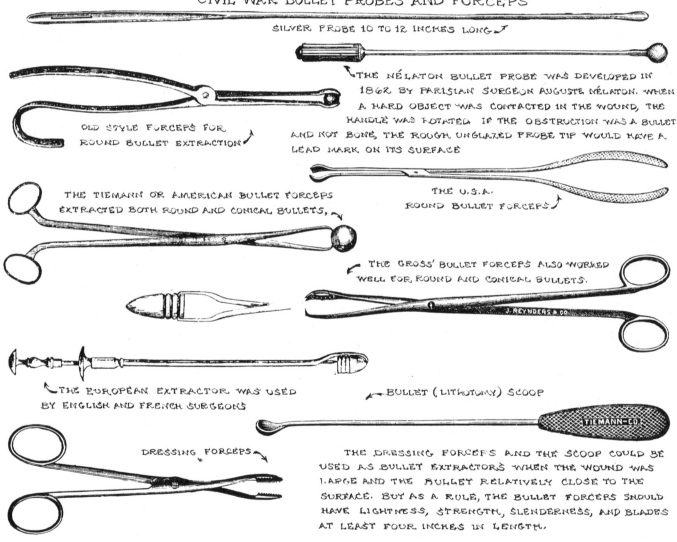

SILVER PROBE 10 TO 12 INCHES LONG.

THE NÉLATON BULLET PROBE WAS DEVELOPED IN 1862 BY PARISIAN SURGEON AUGUSTE NÉLATON. WHEN A HARD OBJECT WAS CONTACTED IN THE WOUND, THE HANDLE WAS ROTATED. IF THE OBSTRUCTION WAS A BULLET AND NOT BONE, THE ROUGH UNGLAZED PROBE TIP WOULD HAVE A LEAD MARK ON ITS SURFACE

OLD STYLE FORCEPS FOR ROUND BULLET EXTRACTION

THE TIEMANN OR AMERICAN BULLET FORCEPS EXTRACTED BOTH ROUND AND CONICAL BULLETS.

THE U.S.A. ROUND BULLET FORCEPS

THE GROSS' BULLET FORCEPS ALSO WORKED WELL FOR ROUND AND CONICAL BULLETS.

THE EUROPEAN EXTRACTOR WAS USED BY ENGLISH AND FRENCH SURGEONS

BULLET (LITHOTOMY) SCOOP

DRESSING FORCEPS

THE DRESSING FORCEPS AND THE SCOOP COULD BE USED AS BULLET EXTRACTORS WHEN THE WOUND WAS LARGE AND THE BULLET RELATIVELY CLOSE TO THE SURFACE. BUT AS A RULE, THE BULLET FORCEPS SHOULD HAVE LIGHTNESS, STRENGTH, SLENDERNESS, AND BLADES AT LEAST FOUR INCHES IN LENGTH.

Any bullet beyond the finger's reach might be located with a metal probe. Since injured vessels may have contracted and begun clotting, careless probing could start a hemorrhage. Once the bullet and any other foreign bodies carried along with it were located, bullet forceps or a scoop were used for its removal. All that was then needed was a dressing of moistened lint covered with oiled silk to prevent evaporation. Now it would be up to the healthy soldier's white blood cells to engulf the bacteria and form pus that, with luck, would drain out the bullet's pathway while recuperating at the regimental or general hospital.

The more severe the injury the more profound the patient's shock. Internal bleeding from a bullet in the chest or abdomen caused the deepest collapse, usually with a fatal outcome. Telltale signs were the pale face that was pinched and anxious, a weak voice, cold hands and feet, a thready pulse that might well be irregular and fluttering, and then a coma that would end in death. Because opening these body cavities was out of the question, the soldier must have strict bed rest with head lowered for a better cerebral blood supply, be given stimulants, and provided with warmth to the extremities. The surgeon hoped that the depressed state might permit clotting of the internal bleeding short of death (see Sidelight 8).

WOUNDS WITH HEMORRHAGE

Before the Civil War, stemming the flow of blood from a lacerated artery deep in the tissues called for a very skilled or daring surgeon. The massive number of projectile wounds throughout that conflict soon earned the field hospital surgeon both of these qualities. Some lesser hemorrhages might be controlled by nothing more than finger pressure over the proximal part of the vessel or into the wound itself— directly on the lacerated wall. Or a tourniquet could control more extensive bleeding by compressing the artery against a bone. In any case, the circular elastic and the middle muscle fiber layer of all arteries contracted on injury. The added pressure helped the laceration to close and seal itself with clotting.

FIELD U.S.A. TOURNIQUET

Another aid to lessen bleeding problems was the use of local styptics: chemical irritants like silver nitrate that could be applied to the torn vessel to speed contraction and clot formation. If an arm or a leg were involved, it could be elevated and cold water applied. The Confederate "Manual of Military Surgery" noted that "opium is the one indispensable drug on the battlefield— important to the surgeon, as gunpowder to the ordinance officer— for besides the ages of pain for which it is the reprieve as an anodyne [pain reliever] it saves rivers of blood as a haemostatic." No doubt this was based on "arterial excitement" being caused by the bullet or saber's "direct inflammation" injury. Perhaps you recall Dr. John Brown's widely accepted theories on page 3.

PETIT'S SCREW TOURNIQUET

If the unwelcomed pulsating spurt of blood should renew after the finger or tourniquet pressure was removed, then the blood vessel should be ligated. Usually the projectile's path must be enlarged by knife and finger retraction. If the artery

DRAWING OUT AND TYING

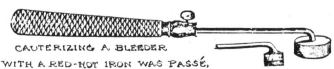

CAUTERIZING A BLEEDER
WITH A RED-HOT IRON WAS PASSÉ.

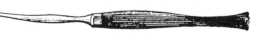

THE SHARP-HOOKED TENACULUM CONTINUED
ITS USEFULNESS THROUGHOUT THE CIVIL WAR.

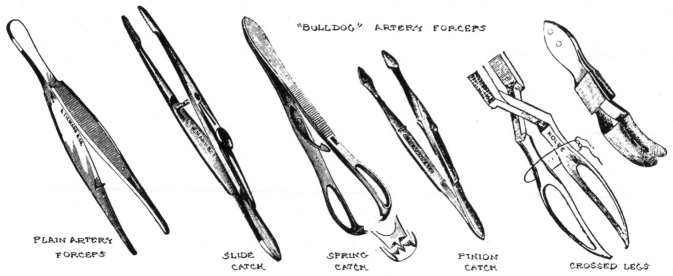

"BULLDOG" ARTERY FORCEPS

PLAIN ARTERY FORCEPS | SLIDE CATCH | SPRING CATCH | PINION CATCH | CROSSED LEGS

MOST BULLDOG FORCEPS WERE DEVELOPED IN THE 1830s. THEY MADE STEADY INROADS ON THE TIME-HONORED TENACULUM DURING THE CIVIL WAR AND PERSISTED INTO THE EARLY 1900s. ALL SHARED THE NAME "BULLDOG" EXCEPT FOR THE PLAIN ARTERY FORCEPS. THEY WERE SELF-LOCKING AND GRIPPED THE ARTERY WITH BULLDOG-LIKE TEETH OR SERRATIONS. THE VARIED CATCHES AND HAVING FENESTRATED OR SOLID JAWS HAD NO BEARING ON THE TERM.

was completely divided, an artery clamp or tenaculum was used to grasp each severed end in turn. A ligature could then be slipped down the instrument and tied. If the lacerated artery wall was still attached, an aneurysm needle could quite handily pass a ligature under each side of the tear for tying. With luck, the collateral circulation would detour around the tied artery by enlarging the arterioles and capillaries in the surrounding tissues.

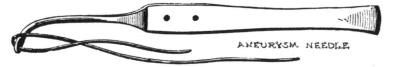

ANEURYSM NEEDLE

For all internal ligatures, absorbable catgut was preferred if available. Otherwise silk or linen ties would do if one end of each deep stitch remained long enough to extend out of the wound. A blood clot should have formed behind the tie in three to four days for small vessels and seven to ten days for the larger ones. A gentle tug on the protruding stitch should complete the healing.

But the danger of a life threatening secondary hemorrhage at the sutured site was very real. Considering the unsterilized sutures, bandaging, and the habit of many surgeons to moisten the thread with bacteria-ladened saliva before threading the needle, it was more than possible that an

THE EXTERNAL SUTURES OF THE CIVIL WAR ARE USED TODAY.

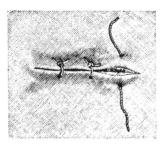

INTERRUPTED SUTURE

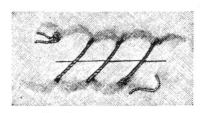

CONTINUOUS SUTURE

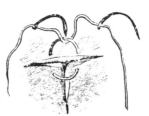

DOUBLE-NEEDLED SUTURE

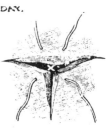

CROSS SUTURE

infection would prevent an adequate clot formation. Then a pull on the protuding suture could bring on a secondary hemorrhage disaster and death.

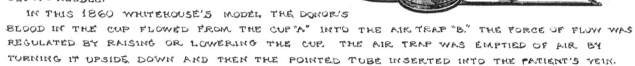

BLOOD TRANSFUSIONS WERE IN THEIR INFANCY AND POORLY UNDERSTOOD AT THIS TIME. TRANSFUSIONS WERE ATTEMPTED JUST TWICE DURING THE CIVIL WAR. ONE PATIENT SURVIVED AND THE OTHER DIED, PERHAPS FROM AN INCOMPATIBLE BLOOD TYPE OR A SEPTIC NEEDLE.

IN THIS 1860 WHITEHOUSE'S MODEL THE DONOR'S BLOOD IN THE CUP FLOWED FROM THE CUP "A" INTO THE AIR TRAP "B." THE FORCE OF FLOW WAS REGULATED BY RAISING OR LOWERING THE CUP. THE AIR TRAP WAS EMPTIED OF AIR BY TURNING IT UPSIDE DOWN AND THEN THE POINTED TUBE INSERTED INTO THE PATIENT'S VEIN.

The relatively few sabre slashes were usually aimed at the head or upper extremities, while the bayonet usually targeted the chest and abdomen resulting in a higher mortality rate. As for bullets and other projectiles, they could penetrate any part of the body and caused well over 99 percent of all Civil War wounds (see Sidelight 9).

WOUNDS OF THE HEAD

A superficial scalp wound needed little more than a covering of moist lint, a spare diet, and rest unless the almost inevitable "laudable pus" began to extend beyond the injury. But a real field hospital emergency was at hand when a soldier presented himself with a depressed skull fracture under a lacerated scalp. The wound must be enlarged and any bone fragments elevated or removed from the brain surface. Only if a bullet were in easy reach in the brain tissue would it be extracted.

A skull fracture also had a real potential for developing an abscess between the dura mater ~ that fibrous wrapping about the brain ~ and the cracked skull that encased it. This would be a general hospital problem and not for the field hospital, for symptoms would not develop until fifteen to thirty days after the injury. It was an ominous finding.

The practice of trephining the skull for any gunshot wound to the head had largely disappeared by the time of the Civil War. Boring such a hole would be indicated only for the presence of a subdural abscess, a growing hematoma, or a slightly depressed fracture that was leading to a permanent dysfunction. Time would reveal these problems after such patients had been sent from the field hospital to the general hospital for recovery and observation. And

"MILITARY SURGEON'S MEDICAL INSTRUMENT BAG, OFTEN CARRIED ON THE FIELD OF BATTLE." GETTYSBURG NATIONAL MILITARY PARK

since trephining carried with it a 61 percent mortality in the Union hospitals it was not a procedure to be taken lightly.

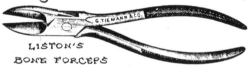

FIELD HOSPITAL, BATTLE OF BRISTOE STATION, VIRGINIA OCTOBER 12-14, 1863

WOUNDS OF THE CHEST

A spent bullet might do little more than bruise the ribs, but a penetrating bullet could shatter that bony cage and puncture the pleural lining. The outside positive pressure would then enter the bullet's pathway and collapse the lung on that side. The patient's shortness of breath and the dullness to percussion when tapping the fingers on the chest wall would give proof of its deflation. If the missile penetrated into the lung tissue, bloody expectoration and a frothy air-and-blood mixture oozing from the wound would be the likely symptoms. The prognosis was poor if the bullet had not exited the chest.

With any chest wound the field hospital surgeon's immediate concern was to ligate any bleeding arteries and remove any rib splinters that might further puncture the air sacks of the lungs. Lint under a broad chest bandage, perfect rest, a dose of opium, and perhaps a short prayer might improve the poor prognosis (the mortality rate for chest wounds was 62 percent). If all went well the air sacks would seal themselves off and re-expand the lung. Because the dictum of that day held that no repair or union of the body could take place unless inflammation and its laudable pus followed, these signs were considered favorable. The development of pleurisy or pneumonia would certainly be life threatening.

LISTON'S BONE FORCEPS

A wound to the heart or one of the major chest arteries was beyond any surgical intervention. The soldier's death would have taken but a few minutes on the battlefield.

"DYING AS AN UNKNOWN ON THE BATTLEFIELD WAS A DREAD THAT LEAD MANY A SOLDIER TO WEAR SOME MEANS OF IDENTIFICATION. FOR SOME, A PIECE OF PAPER PINNED ON THE UNIFORM WITH HIS NAME AND THAT OF A FAMILY MEMBER TO BE NOTIFIED WAS GOOD ENOUGH. OTHERS PURCHASED A MORE ENDURING PENDANT AS SHOWN HERE OR A GOOD LUCK COIN WITH A PATRIOTIC MOTIF ON ONE SIDE AND HIS I.D. ON THE REVERSE. IT WAS NOT UNTIL WORLD WAR I THAT THE UNITED STATES MILITARY ISSUED DOG TAGS TO ITS FIGHTING MEN." GETTYSBURG NATIONAL MILITARY PARK

Z. PETTIT N.Y.V. BRIG.

WOUNDS OF THE ABDOMEN

The abdomen had no such bony armor as the skull or rib cage. A wound to that exposed part would find the soldier in profound shock on admission to the field hospital. Even if he rallied, death from peritonitis would follow. Penetration of the intestine, bladder, abdominal aorta, and like structures would speed the patient into an almost inevitable fate. The mortality rate was no less than 87 percent from these injuries.

WOUNDS OF THE EXTREMITIES

While the salvage from head, chest, and abdominal wounds was less than encouraging, at least primary amputations of the extremities ~ those done within twenty-four hours of being wounded ~ could save lives. After that time inflammation would begin in the wound, likely followed by gangrene and death. With one's life in the balance, the cost of losing a limb didn't seem too high.

We should repeat that the Civil War surgeon would not learn about the germ theory until at least twenty years into the ? future. Therefore he provided a real infection threat above and beyond the battlefield contamination. Dr. W. W. Keen, the well-known Civil War and World War 1 surgeon, remarked that it was seven times safer to fight through the three-day Gettysburg battles than to have a limb amputation or a compound fracture under Civil War surgery.* The diary of General Carl Schurz, commander of the 11th Union Corps at Gettysburg, summed up the septic surgery during that battle:

> "Most of the operating tables were placed in the open where the light was best, some of them partially protected against the rain. There stood the surgeons, their sleeves rolled up to the elbows, their bare arms as well as their linen aprons smeared with blood, their knives not seldom held between their teeth while they were helping the patient on and off the table or had their hands otherwise occupied. Around them pools of blood and amputated arms or legs in heaps sometimes more than a man high."

Well over 70 percent of all projectile wounds involved arms, thighs, legs, hands, and feet. The field surgeon was regarded as an amputation specialist. He must remove any damaged limb that might permit inflammation to

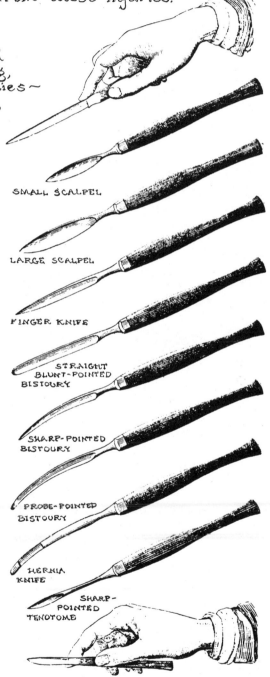

SMALL SCALPEL

LARGE SCALPEL

FINGER KNIFE

STRAIGHT BLUNT-POINTED BISTOURY

SHARP-POINTED BISTOURY

PROBE-POINTED BISTOURY

HERNIA KNIFE

SHARP-POINTED TENOTOME

SEE PAGE 14 FOR THEIR USES.

---

* WHILE HALF OF ALL THE SOLDIERS UNDERGOING AMPUTATIONS DIED AFTER SURGERY, TWO OUT OF THREE WOUNDED SUCCUMBED TO COMPOUND FRACTURES. INFECTION WAS GENERALLY THE CAUSE.

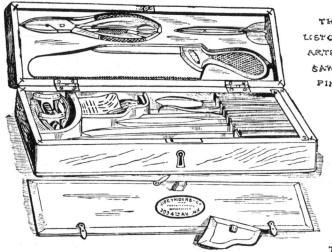

THIS AMPUTATION CASE CONTAINS A LISTON'S LONG KNIFE, LISTON'S MEDIUM KNIFE, CATLING, SCALPEL, TENACULUM, ARTERY FORCEPS, METACARPAL SAW, LARGE MOVABLE BACK SAW, TOURNIQUET, BONE FORCEPS, ONE DOZEN NEEDLES, WAX, PINS, AND SILK SUTURE THREAD.

OUR INSTRUMENT PICTURES THROUGHOUT THIS BOOK ARE TAKEN FROM VARIOUS NINETEENTH CENTURY MEDICAL CATALOGS. FOR TWENTY YEARS AFTER THE CIVIL WAR, THE SURGICAL INSTRUMENTS WERE BASICALLY UNCHANGED. AFTER THAT TIME THEY WERE MADE OF NICKEL-PLATED METAL TO WITHSTAND STERILIZATION SINCE THE ELECTROPLATING OF NICKEL WAS NOT INVENTED UNTIL 1868 BY WILLIAM H. REMINGTON OF BOSTON, MASSACHUSETTS. THEREFORE ALL SURGICAL INSTRUMENTS USED IN THE CIVIL WAR WOULD BE UNPLATED.

extend from the wound to the rest of the body. The indications for the primary amputation were all compound long bone fractures, all bullet wounds to a joint and any fractures that entered the joint, uncontrolled hemorrhage, irreparable lacerations of major blood vessels or nerves, severe lacerations and crushing of tissue, and foreign bodies that were too deep or difficult to remove.

At the outset the surgeon would reassure the patient while the amputation site was being shaved. As the anesthetic was being given, he would make one last check to see that his amputation equipment (tourniquets, amputating knives and saws, artery forceps and tenacula, bone forceps, sponges, and threaded curved needles) was all in readiness and handy on a tray. The tourniquet would be positioned so that its pad would compress the main artery against an underlying bone. Its band was then snugged above the operation site, buckled tightly, and the tourniquet screw tightened. All was in readiness to begin a circular, oval, or flap amputation.

THE CIRCULAR AMPUTATION~

The long, single-edged blade of the amputation knife was swept around perpendicular to the limb, cutting down through the skin, fat, and fascia. While an assistant retracted the proximal

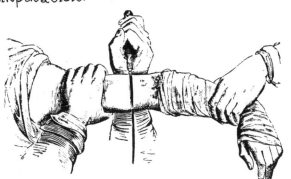

THE DOUBLE-EDGED CATLING WAS BASICALLY A FLAP AMPUTATION INSTRUMENT. IT PENETRATED EASILY THROUGH THE DEPTH OF MUSCLE, THEN COULD CUT IN ANY DIRECTION.

skin of this incised circle, the surgeon made another circular knife sweep close to the retracted skin edge and down through the musculature to the bone(s). The retraction of the skin

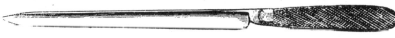

LISTON'S SMALL AMPUTATION KNIFE

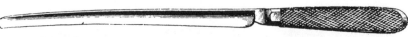

WOOD'S CIRCULAR AMPUTATION KNIFE

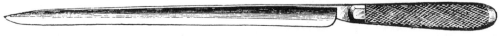

THE SINGLE-EDGED LONG LISTON AMPUTATION KNIFE WAS USED FOR ALL CIRCULAR AND SOMETIMES THE FLAP AMPUTATIONS

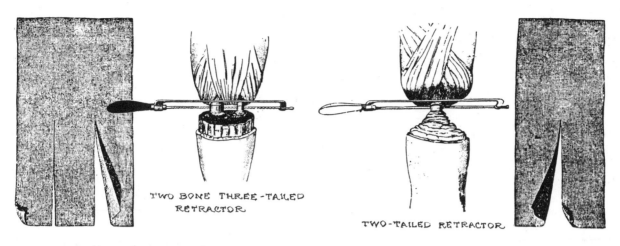

TWO BONE THREE-TAILED RETRACTOR

TWO-TAILED RETRACTOR

gave a hollowed cone of muscle around the bone(s). With the tip of the knife, an inch or two of muscle was freed from the bony surface.

The skin and its underlying musculature must be retracted to permit the bone(s) to be sawn under the released inch or so of muscle. An assistant could use either his hands or a linen cloth retractor for drawing the tissue upward. A single upper arm or leg long bone would need a single slit in the cloth to give two tails. The two lower arm or leg long bones required a three-tailed cloth retractor with the center strip being inserted between the bones. The amputation saw could then reach high on the bone to the apex of the coned muscle and give a decent amount of skin and muscle to cover the stump. A perpendicular cut across the bone was made with the saw and any irregular edges then trimmed and smoothed with a "rongeur" (gnawing forceps).

With the retractors removed, the main arteries could be identified. The vessels were drawn out with artery forceps or hooked out with a tenaculum. Each was tied with a ligature. The tourniquet was then loosened to identify lesser arteries that still bled and were in want of tying. Before ligating any artery, accompanying nerves must be separated and not tied with the vessel or else painful neuralgia would forever plague the patient. Veins generally

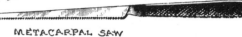

METACARPAL SAW

LIFTING-BACK METACARPAL SAW
METACARPAL SAWS AMPUTATED THE HAND BONES TO THE WRIST AS WELL AS ANY SMALLER DIAMETER LONG BONES.

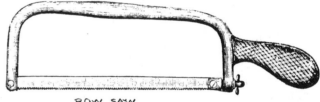

BOW SAW

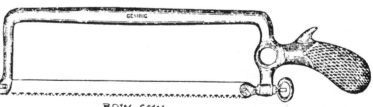

BOW SAW

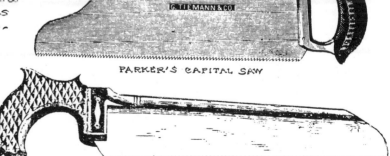

G. TIEMANN & CO.

PARKER'S CAPITAL SAW

THE CAPITAL AMPUTATION SAW SEVERED THE LARGER LONG BONES.

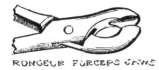

RONGEUR FORCEPS JAWS

collapse and clot, but if any persisted in oozing, finger pressure and raising the limb usually stopped any bleeding. If not the vein must be tied or cauterized. All nonabsorbable silk or linen ligatures should have one end long enough to hang out of the stump when the skin edges were brought together. As noted under "HEMORRHAGE," the ties would be free in a week or so of healing and could usually be removed. Much to be preferred, when available, were the self-absorbing catgut ligatures whenever suturing or ligating was needed within the body.

The stump was then cleaned and the skin and muscle pulled down and over the end of the bone. The edges of the skin could then be brought together and strapped in position with a strip of adhesive plaster.* No skin sutures were usually necessary. Spaces were left for any long nonabsorbable ligature ends and for any drainage. Lint or cotton, held in place by a bandage, absorbed any drainage during the period of healing.

THE FLAP AMPUTATION ~ Since prehistoric times the circular amputation had been the only way to remove part of a limb. Then in 1837 Robert Liston popularized the flap amputation, which understandably gained favor. The method was considered faster, gave more skin coverage to the stump and better approximation than the circular cut, and gave less postoperative pain. The preparation for the operation, use of the tourniquet and saw, ligation of vessels and dressings were much the same as those found in the foregoing circular amputation description.

The Single Flap amputation was designed for amputations below the knee. An oblique incision was first made through the skin and subcutaneous tissue from the base of the calf proximally over the the tibia and fibula. After retraction the underlying tissue was cut to the bone, leaving the gastrocnemius muscle for padding the stump. It was also called the Oval Amputation because of its oblique cut.

SINGLE FLAP

After retraction and sawing of the bone(s), the flap was brought forward. Since the flap was large and bulky, it was prudent to approximate the skin edges with interrupted sutures about an inch apart. The inevitable inflammation process that followed could drain the purulent matter. Metallic sutures of thin wire were preferred because of their holding power, but silk thread made a reasonable substitute. Adhesive plaster strips helped to approximate any wayward skin edges.

DOUBLE FLAP

The Double Flap amputation began with the surgeon grasping and raising the anterior skin and muscles from the bone(s). The point of the amputation knife was pushed horizontally through the side of the limb until it encountered the bone. The point was then guided UP AND OVER, then through the muscle beyond until it exited through the skin opposite its entrance. The blade was then angled upward and distally to give an anterior flap. The knife was reinserted into the

* IN 1845 IT WAS FOUND THAT RUBBER COULD BE CHANGED TO A GUMMY LIQUID WHEN DISSOLVED IN A SOLVENT SUCH AS BENZENE AND TURPENTINE. IT WAS SPREAD ON CLOTH, AND THE STICKY SURFACE BECAME THE MUCH-USED ADHESIVE PLASTER IN THE CIVIL WAR.

initial opening and along the same course until again meeting the bone(s). This time the point was worked UNDER and then slightly upward until the previous exit was reached and the blade angled downward to match the first flap. As the assistants gradually retracted the flaps, the surgeon severed any tissue that remained in the angle between the flaps. The bone could then be sawn free and the skin and muscle drawn forward to join the two skin edges by interrupted sutures and adhesive plaster strips (see Sidelight 10).

FRACTURES

Fractures were no strangers to the battlefield, and there were many that did not demand the drastic amputation procedures of a contaminated compound fracture. Such were those bone breaks that didn't perforate the skin, the simple fractures. Most would serve the soldier well in the days to come unless rough handling on the litter or ambulance converted a simple fracture to a compound one. Temporary splinting at the ambulance depot or first aid station would guard the limb until the field hospital was reached.

A simple fracture might be nothing more worrisome than a transverse crack. The more severe greenstick fracture was partly broken and partly intact. It was still fairly stable in spite of the deformity and limb-shortening that were apparent on examination. Worse yet was a completely severed long bone from a blow or projectile, which was unstable. The field hospital surgeon could locate any displacement from its shortening and the grating sound and feeling when the broken ends rub together. It might well be fragmented~ that is, a comminuted fracture~ if struck by shot or a bullet. Because progressive pain, swelling, and intertissue bleeding would soon mask the full extent of the fracture and increase muscle spasm to make any reduction of a displaced bone difficult, the surgeon would make his examination as soon as possible.

The skin would be washed to help prevent perspiration that would cause itching after splinting. The greenstick and displaced fractures must be straightened with the broken edges again joined. Usually an assistant held the extremity above the fracture while the surgeon drew the overriding or bent lower part away from the body. He might use firm hand pressure to better align the long bone or manipulate the shattered pieces of a comminuted fracture into better position. Generally two wooden splints were applied, one for each side of a limb. The less stable

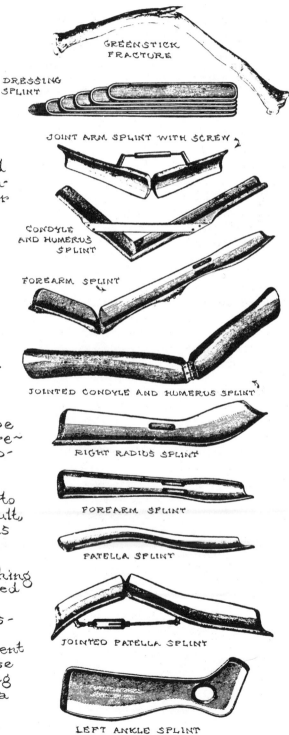

GREENSTICK FRACTURE

DRESSING SPLINT

JOINT ARM SPLINT WITH SCREW

CONDYLE AND HUMERUS SPLINT

FOREARM SPLINT

JOINTED CONDYLE AND HUMERUS SPLINT

RIGHT RADIUS SPLINT

FOREARM SPLINT

PATELLA SPLINT

JOINTED PATELLA SPLINT

LEFT ANKLE SPLINT

CARVED HARDWOOD SPLINTS

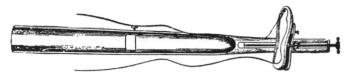

EXTENSION BAR FOR LEG FRACTURE REDUCTION

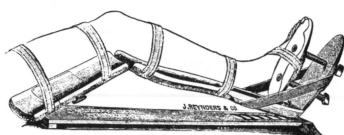

DOUBLE INCLINE PLANE LEG SPLINT

J. REYNDERS & CO.

fracture of a thigh bone deserved traction in addition to the two splints that ran the length of the leg.

There were three ways to secure a splint or splints to a fractured bone: 1. The looped bandage was a series of folded cloth strips no more than 3 inches apart that bound the splints. One end of each tie was left longer to tie to its neighboring loop. This had the advantage of loosening if swelling around the break was impeding circulation. 2. The tailed

bandage was one with each tail overlapping the previous tail (see page 40). It gave a snug hold to the splints but could not be loosened or tightened. 3. The common roller bandage was the easiest and simplest of all but used only where the fracture was fairly stable and the roller could be carried under the splinting without endangering the reduction. (Also see page 40 for the figure of 8 roller bandage for a fractured clavicle). At the first sign of blue or numb fingers or toes, the bandages must be loosened to improve the blood flow blocked by swollen tissues.

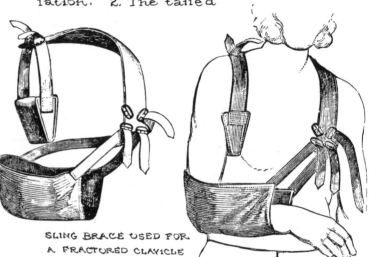

SLING BRACE USED FOR A FRACTURED CLAVICLE

HOSPITAL TRAINS

When a wounded soldier left the field hospital by ambulance, he might be returned to the regimental hospital if his condition permitted and if his regiment was not in the field on campaign. For those with more extensive surgery and possible postoperative complications, recuperation would be at a general hospital. For those hospitals one hundred or more miles away, the transportation of choice would be the railroad. But there were problems. At the beginning of the war the Federal government had granted contracts to private railroads for carrying the casualties to the general hospitals. Any care or comfort provided by those for-profit companies was little more than box cars strewn with hay ~ along with the unmistakable aroma of previous patients with intestinal complaints. Although little is known of the Confederate rail removal of patients, their early efforts in the war also were likely hobbled by inexperience.

Fortunately for the Union troops, the Sanitary Commission watchdogs were well aware of such discomforts plaguing the wounded. In the summer of 1862, the United States completed the military takeover of the Northern rail lines. That fall Dr. Elisha Harris planned and supervised the outfitting and conversion of sleeping cars into hospital cars. Each severely wounded patient was brought directly to the train on a stretcher. Pain, exertion, and complications such as sudden wound hemorrhage or fracture displacement from the rough treatment of earlier days were now more of a rarity.

Each stretcher had large rubber rings attached to the four handles. Once aboard, the rings would be hung on hooks secured into wooden support posts. The stretcher and its patient were suspended on one of the three tiers in the 50-foot hospital car. There was one small glitch. The elastic rubber bands vibrated the stretchers when the train was in motion. The rigs were called "capering beds" by their occupants but still were pure luxury when compared to the slow torture of box car and hay.

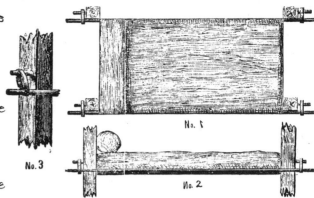

THE "HARRIS CAR" RUBBER RING SUSPENSION OF LITTERS: 1. VERTICAL VIEW; 2. LATERAL VIEW; 3. AN ENLARGED VIEW OF THE RUBBER RINGS.

PASSENGER RAILROAD CAR FITTED UP AS A HOSPITAL CAR.

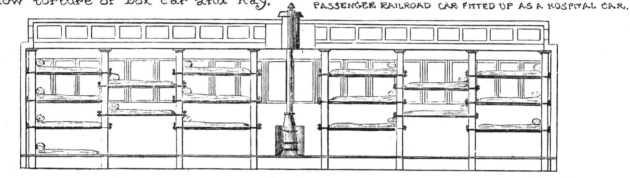

By fall the new hospital cars were making regular daily runs between Washington and New York with comfortable beds, a proper diet, and skilled care. This was progress indeed but not soon enough for the staggering number of casualties from the great battle of Gettysburg. Fortunately Dr. Letterman's innovative ambulance corps was able to remove all of the wounded from the battlefield by the end of each day. Although the trains of box cars had to make do, three-quarters of the field hospital patients were on their way to the general hospitals in just two weeks. It was all the more remarkable because the Gettysburg railroad branch had been destroyed and had to first be rebuilt before trains could service the area.

The Gettysburg victory on July 3, 1863, and the surrender the following day of Vicksburg

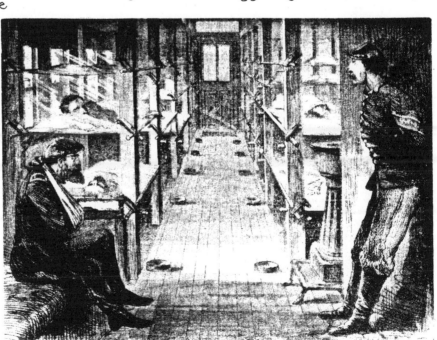

INTERIOR OF THE CONVERTED HOSPITAL CAR

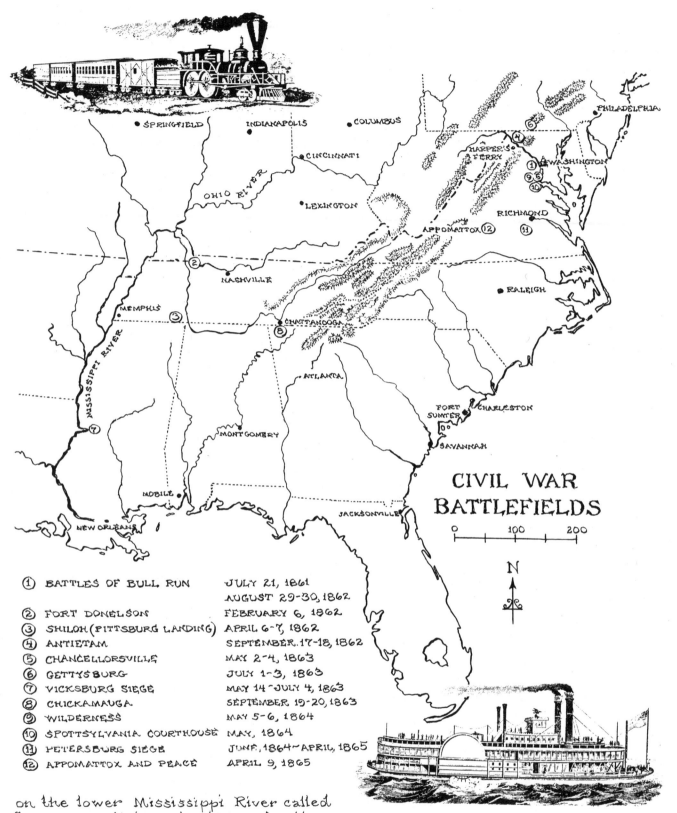

CIVIL WAR BATTLEFIELDS

0	100	200		

N

① BATTLES OF BULL RUN   JULY 21, 1861
                                    AUGUST 29-30, 1862
② FORT DONELSON   FEBRUARY 6, 1862
③ SHILOH (PITTSBURG LANDING)   APRIL 6-7, 1862
④ ANTIETAM   SEPTEMBER 17-18, 1862
⑤ CHANCELLORSVILLE   MAY 2-4, 1863
⑥ GETTYSBURG   JULY 1-3, 1863
⑦ VICKSBURG SIEGE   MAY 14-JULY 4, 1863
⑧ CHICKAMAUGA   SEPTEMBER 19-20, 1863
⑨ WILDERNESS   MAY 5-6, 1864
⑩ SPOTTSYLVANIA COURTHOUSE   MAY, 1864
⑪ PETERSBURG SIEGE   JUNE, 1864-APRIL, 1865
⑫ APPOMATTOX AND PEACE   APRIL 9, 1865

on the lower Mississippi River called
for a new Union strategy. As the
Army of the Potomac pressed southward toward Richmond, the Army of the
Cumberland drove eastward from their Mississippi River bases, following the
main rail line between Nashville and Chattanooga in Tennessee and on to
Georgia. As the Army of the Cumberland advanced, the captured rail was
used to bring in munitions and supplies. The return trip brought the new

ambulance trains and their wounded the distance back to the various general hospitals.

The usual hospital train carried between five and ten hospital cars, a surgeon's car, a passenger car with seats for any soldier not confined to bed, a kitchen car, and probably a box car with supplies. The staff of the surgeon-in-charge included a medical assistant and a hospital steward along with enlisted nurses, hospital attendants, and cooks. These special trains announced themselves with U.S. HOSPITAL TRAIN painted in large letters on the car panels and the yellow flag on the engine. In the dark of night, three red lanterns were hung under the headlight of the engine. The train would run at a comfortably low speed with up to two hundred patients in the larger ten-car hospital train.

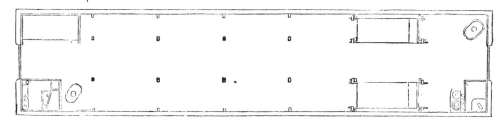

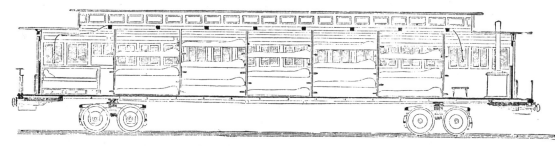

HOSPITAL RAILWAY CAR USED IN THE EAST

Meanwhile the hardships suffered by the Confederate wounded were being multiplied. The Union blockade that crippled the inflow of arms and munitions also reduced supplies of anesthetics and medications. The hard-worked Southern railway system was wearing out. The lack of rail replacements to carry troops to the front also meant that casualties on the return had problems reaching their general hospitals for convalescence. Private J.B. Roden of the 7th Louisiana Regiment wrote of his efforts to reach the Winder General Hospital:

"I was wounded on the skirmish line May 18, 1864. I passed to the field hospital where the doctor examined my wounds and told me he would have to perform an operation. When I asked if amputation would be necessary, he said 'Not just now.' This was not very comforting as it left the impression it might be later.

"The operating table was a barn door set on two trestles. When chloroform was administered, it was reported the patient sang 'The Bonny Blue Flag' and other war songs.

"Immediately after the operation it was reported that Grant's Army had turned our right flank and captured Guinea Station; consequently all wounded were ordered to the rear. All who could walk were ordered to do so, the nearest station being Milford, some 30 miles distant. I started alone about 2 p.m., the sun being near full and made 12 miles, stopping at a farmhouse overnight where I was treated very kindly. Having yet 18 miles before me, I started early and made 14 miles when I fell exhausted by the roadside. I was put on a wagon and hauled to the station four miles over a country road. There I was put on a hospital train, remaining all night at the station and arrived at Richmond the next evening, where I was taken to (Winder) hospital, this being Friday afternoon. On Sunday morning the surgeon in charge, Dr. Tyler, examined and dressed my wound, nothing having been done to it since Wednesday, except the use of cold water to keep down the inflammation.*

HOSPITAL SHIPS

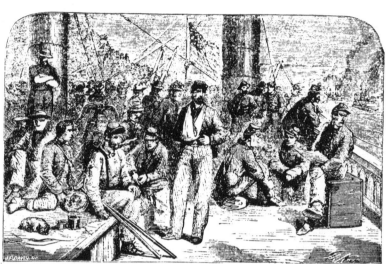

MISSISSIPPI RIVER HOSPITAL STEAMER

Supplies were being shipped to General McClellan's Peninsula Campaign on whatever rough and rusty freighters that could be requisitioned. The United States Sanitary Commission had considered the quandary of piled-up Union casualties along the Chesapeake Bay shores and the possibilities of converting some of those old steamers for hospital ship duty. Early in the spring of 1862, the Commission was able to convince the Medical Department and the quartermaster general to convert some of these seagoing veterans for hospital duty: small boats could ferry the casualties down the many rivers and creeks along the Chesapeake to the waiting vessels.

The Commission was assigned a weathered old veteran, the "Daniel Webster," that was berthed at Alexandria and said to be "stripped of everything but dirt." Under the direction of Frederick Law Olmsted, the ship was refurbished. In April 1862 she steamed for the battle zone as the first hospital ship of the eastern coast. She carried a complement of six medical students, twenty volunteer male nurses, four ladies

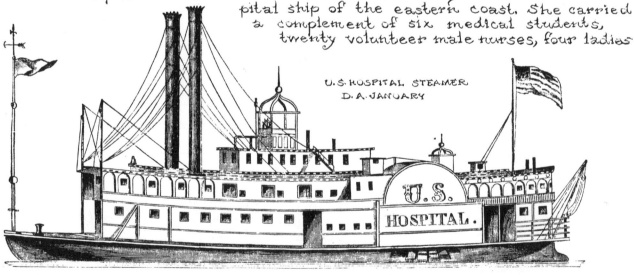

U.S. HOSPITAL STEAMER
D. A. JANUARY

* TO UPDATE PRIVATE RODEN'S HOSPITALIZATION, HIS STAY WORE ON FOR EIGHT WEEKS BECAUSE HIS ARM WOUND BECAME INFECTED. ALTHOUGH "STILL UNABLE TO REACH MY MOUTH WITH THAT SHATTERED ARM," IT WAS ALSO BEYOND REACH OF THE SURGEON'S KNIFE.

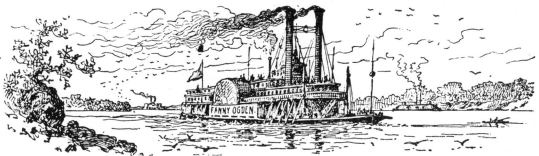

THE MISSISSIPPI STEAMER "FANNY OGDEN" ON HER WAY FOR ANOTHER CARGO OF SICK AND WOUNDED UNION SOLDIERS.

to assist (but without cumbersome hoops in their dresses), five Commission members, eight military officers, and ninety convalescent soldiers returning to their regiments ~ all in addition to the ship's hands.

The military police were aboard to maintain army discipline and to permit aboard only those patients certified to be unfit for duty within thirty days. The Commission supervised all shipboard administration and the care and comfort of the wounded. They brought touches of home to the patients: homemade jellies, molasses, and fresh bread, "nice thick soup," rice pudding, lemonade, milk punch, black tea ~ preferred to green tea ~ oranges, as well as wine and brandy. There were also fresh towels, handkerchiefs, cologne, bed sacks filled with fresh straw, blankets, and, best of all, conversations with real live volunteer ladies.

Grant's offensive down the Mississippi River was under way in 1862, and the Union navy had scooped up the larger river steamers. They were converted to gunboats with armored hulls. The western branch of the Sanitary Commission was able to lease several smaller vessels. The first was the "City of Memphis" at Fort Henry in February, followed by the "Hazel Dell," "Franklin," "War Eagle," and "City of Louisiana." Rentals drained most of the available funds, but in the pinch civilians such as one feisty volunteer nurse, "Mother" Byckerdyke (who deserves a separate book about her bucking deadhead brass and cutting through red tape), came through with the needed supplies and equipment to carry over seven thousand casualties, Yankee and Rebel, to the Ohio River hospitals.

General Grant's advance down the Mississippi River captured "Island Number Ten" on April 7 and netted four Confederate steamers. One of these, the "Red Rover," had been damaged by mortar fire. After

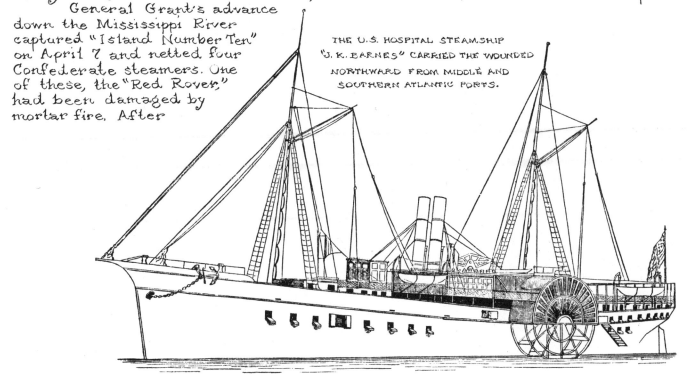

THE U.S. HOSPITAL STEAMSHIP "J. K. BARNES" CARRIED THE WOUNDED NORTHWARD FROM MIDDLE AND SOUTHERN ATLANTIC PORTS.

being floated to Cairo and made riverworthy once again, it began its new life as the first official United States Navy hospital ship. The restoration was under the guidance of the United States Sanitary Commission. By June 10 this "floating palace," as she was called, cast off to pick up her first load of hospital-bound soldiers. The ship had elevators between decks, an advanced operating room, screened ports, and, as Admiral Porter of the Mississippi squadron said, it was "fitted with every comfort, and poor Jack, when sick or wounded, was cared for in a style never before dreamed of in the Navy."

THE ARMY GENERAL HOSPITAL

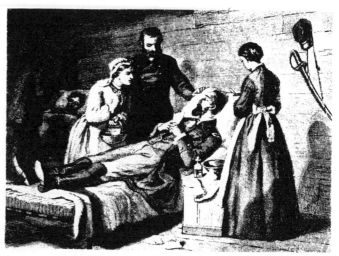

As far as the average pre-Civil War citizen was concerned, a hospital would be one of the sights to see on a trip to the big city. But back in the village, folks had their sick times at home. Only the town's almshouse occasionally acted as a hospital for the indigent. That was before the Battle of Bull Run became a wake-up call for a better way to treat those wounded who needed long-term care.

A military general hospital was the answer, and its guidelines were founded back in the Revolutionary War. Camp contagions were found to have less of a chance to spread when the soldiers were hospitalized in separate buildings~ uncrowded, well ventilated, and with attention paid to cleanliness and decent food. The British medics in the Crimean War followed a similar plan for what was known as pavilioned hospitals. Covered pavilion walkways with fresh air circulating freely through the open sides connected each separate building.

Each of these long, low wards hosted between sixty and one hundred patients. Each would have a ventilated roof to remove any inflammation-carrying noxious vapors, an uncluttered interior for easier cleaning and white-washing, and up-to-date garbage and sewage disposal.

Both Northern and Southern armies were hardly aware that the early makeshift hotels, factories, churches,

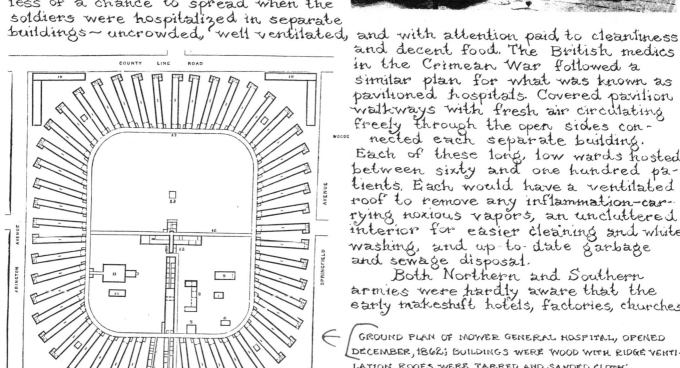

GROUND PLAN OF MOWER GENERAL HOSPITAL, OPENED DECEMBER, 1862; BUILDINGS WERE WOOD WITH RIDGE VENTILATION, ROOFS WERE TARRED AND SANDED CLOTH:

1 WARDS; 2 RECEPTION ROOM, LAUNDRY, ETC.; KITCHEN BETWEEN 2 AND 12; 3 KNAPSACK AND BAND ROOM; 4 STOREROOMS; 5 OPERATING ROOMS; 6 BUTCHER'S SHOP; 7 GUARD HOUSE, 8 BOILERS, COAL; 9 SUTLER; 10 CARPENTER; 11 CHAPEL; 12 ADMINISTRATION; 13 ICEHOUSE; 14,15, RAILROAD DEPOTS; 16,17, CORRIDORS; 18 BARRACKS.

warehouses ~ and even General Robert E. Lee's mansion across the Potomac then being used for the Union wounded ~ were not the answer for healing the many in a long-term, all-out war. Changing Washington's mind-set was no easy chore. It took the collective heads of the United States Sanitary Commission and Dr. William Hammond, then inspector of hospitals at Wheeling, to sell the general hospital idea.

In Rebel country Surgeon General Dr. Samuel Moore could squeeze but $50,000 from a tightfisted Confederate Congress for pavilion hospitals. Many general hospitals, as in the North, required little more than a roof to earn that name. No matter. Moore moved ahead with his plans, and by October 1861 he had opened the Chimborazo pavilion hospital at Richmond ~ the largest of the entire war. The size of a small town and serviced by the Confederate capital's five rail lines, the hospital could boast of thirty separate ward buildings of 30 by 100 feet in size, each holding sixty patients. The patients were served by five kitchens, a bakery, five ice houses, bath houses, a laundry, a 400-keg-capacity brewery, and even its own boats that could sail along the James River to collect food. Other noteworthy pavilion hospitals on not as grand a scale were Howard's Grove and Winder general hospitals.

Chimborazo's success must have impressed the Confederate Congress, for more funds were found for construction of new or rehabilitated older buildings throughout the South. Being states-rights minded, that governing body made sure that the hospitals were scattered throughout the South. Dr. Samuel H. Stout saw to the new and the older redesigned buildings. By the end of the war, Stout had placed twenty-three army general hospitals, with or without pavilions, in Alabama; four in Florida; fifty in Georgia; three in Mississippi; twenty-one in North Carolina; twelve in South Carolina; two in Tennessee; and thirty-nine in Virginia.

As for the Union's drive to build general pavilion hospitals, the Judiciary Square and Mount Pleasant hospitals were in operation by April 1862. When Hammond replaced Dr. Clement Finley as surgeon general, he made it his business to build state-of-the-art pavilion hospitals throughout the North. When the war was over in 1865, more than 200 such hospitals had been built, with a total of 137,000 beds. They had served over a million patients and lost a surprisingly low number ~ less than 10 percent ~ of hospitalized sick and wounded who died in those presterilization days.

Here follows some of the diagnostic and therapeutic instruments available but little known or used during the Civil War period.

FORMER CONFEDERATE SURGEON SAMUEL H. STOUT

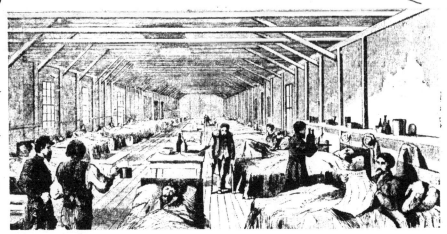

THE UNITED STATES GENERAL HOSPITAL, HILTON HEAD, SOUTH CAROLINA

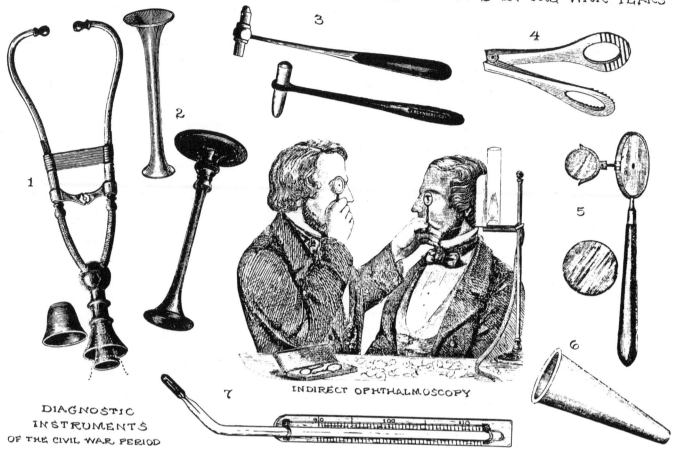

INDIRECT OPHTHALMOSCOPY

DIAGNOSTIC INSTRUMENTS OF THE CIVIL WAR PERIOD

1 Cammann binaural stethoscope, American c.1856, with interchangeable bell chest pieces~post-war Americans preferred it to the monaural stethoscope.

2 The monaural stethoscope was an on-the-spot inspiration of French physician René Laennac in 1816. Too embarrassed to press his ear against the bosom of a well-endowed female patient to hear the heart and lungs, he rolled up a sheaf of paper and listened at a distance. These examples are of turned hardwood with a central hole. The chest ends are smaller than the ear ends. The monaural stethoscopes were recommended to America when Oliver Wendell Holmes returned from his Paris studies in 1835.

3 Flint's percussor, American c.1860, was devised by Dr. Austin Flint to tap the chest for resonance. However he did admit after the Civil War came to a close that physicians still preferred striking their first or second finger against the patient's chest because the percussors were always "at hand."

4 Folding tongue depressor, c.1845, simply hinged the usual metal or wooden flat stick into a convenient space-saving pocket carrier of unplated steel.

5 Liebreich's ophthalmoscope, European c.1855, made direct viewing of the inner eye obsolete. A pivoting arm held either a concave or a convex lens for indirect inspection through a hole in its mirror. Reflected light illuminated the retina. The popularity of the ophthalmoscope grew rapidly after the Civil War.

6 The ear speculum, c.1830, was a simple hollow cone used for viewing the canal and drum with either direct or indirect lighting.

7 The clinical thermometer was fragile, cumbersome, and the patient's temperature was taken from the axilla. The ivory scale was attached and not etched into the glass. Even so, the thermometer found more extensive use in the Civil War than was previously thought (see Sidelight 11).

8 Grunow's large microscope, American c.1853, was but one of many European and American microscopes available. It would find use in the army general hospitals with particular emphasis on pathology.

THERAPEUTIC INSTRUMENTS ~ Until the germ theory could one day make believers of the medical profession, advances in therapy would be less than inspiring. The hypodermic syringe had real promise but like many of the diagnostic innovations it arrived too late on the Civil War scene to be of much use.

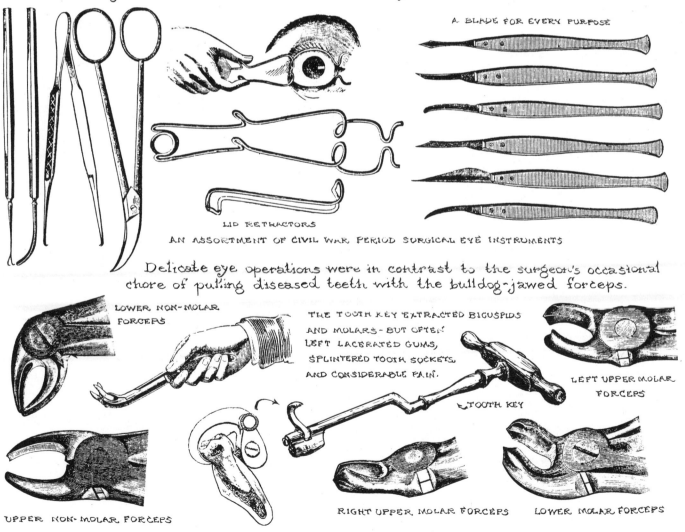

THIS IS THE ORIGINAL HYPODERMIC SYRINGE INVENTED AND USED BY DR. ALEXANDER WOOD OF EDINBURG IN 1853.
MUSEUM OF THE ROYAL COLLEGE OF SURGEONS, LONDON

UNION ARMY LIEUTENANT COLONEL DR. JOHN BILLINGS USED THE FIRST HYPODERMIC SYRINGE AT THE 1862 SEVEN DAYS BATTLE NEAR RICHMOND. NO MORE THAN A DOZEN WERE IN USE BY 1865. THEY PROBABLY RESEMBLED THIS c.1850 HYPODERMIC SYRINGE. WELLCOME HISTORICAL MEDICAL MUSEUM, LONDON

These eye instruments were available to surgeons of considerable skill.

A BLADE FOR EVERY PURPOSE

LID RETRACTORS

AN ASSORTMENT OF CIVIL WAR PERIOD SURGICAL EYE INSTRUMENTS

Delicate eye operations were in contrast to the surgeon's occasional chore of pulling diseased teeth with the bulldog-jawed forceps.

LOWER NON-MOLAR FORCEPS

THE TOOTH KEY EXTRACTED BICUSPIDS AND MOLARS - BUT OFTEN LEFT LACERATED GUMS, SPLINTERED TOOTH SOCKETS, AND CONSIDERABLE PAIN.

LEFT UPPER MOLAR FORCEPS

TOOTH KEY

UPPER NON-MOLAR FORCEPS

RIGHT UPPER MOLAR FORCEPS

LOWER MOLAR FORCEPS

ascites!

Without a doubt field surgeons were the acknowledged specialists for primary amputation, acute hemorrhages, fractures, and other such life-threatening emergencies. By contrast the military general hospitals bedded both acute and chronic medical patients ~ and a broad spectrum of surgery as well. There would be the usual influx of dislocations, burns, aneurysms, pneumothorax, (ascites, hernias, and bladder stones as well as delayed amputations.

Such amputations were intermediary ~ that is, those following the twenty-four-hour primary period and up to and including the onset of the usual inflammation. Secondary amputations were those taking place two or more weeks after the wound and during the formation of pus usually three to six weeks after injury. And finally, reamputations might be necessary if early gangrene had begun in the stump.

Fortunately the general hospital surgeons had the time and luxury to consider the newer surgical techniques. Joint and bone resections had gained recent favor in the world medical circles and among the Civil War casualties as well. By undergoing excision of the diseased soft tissues and the necrotic articulating surfaces of the bones, a soldier need not have his limb amputated. And if a portion of a hard outer cortex or its marrow also suffered destruction from inflammation, that portion could be removed, and the arm or leg, although shortened, would be preserved and useful to the fortunate patient (see Sidelight 12 on hospital supplies).

A choice between resection and amputation would seem a no contest. All major arteries, veins, and nerves would remain intact. No tourniquet was usually needed, and the operation was far less traumatic mentally and physically to the patient. A skilled surgeon, well acquainted with human anatomy and an operating room without the turmoil and stress of the field hospital, could expect to have the soldier whole and carrying on an active life. And if the disease had destroyed too great a part of the extremity to be saved once opened and inspected, amputation could take place without the patient gaining consciousness.

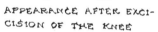

APPEARANCE AFTER EXCISION OF THE KNEE

JOINT RESECTION

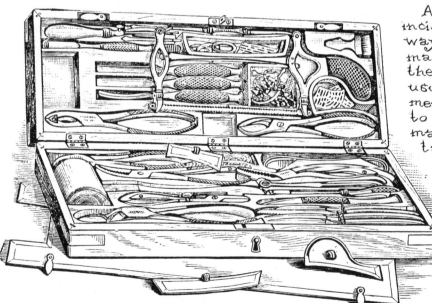

CASED DISECTION INSTRUMENTS

Abscessed joints were often incised along the sinus pathways, those eroded tunnels made by pus escaping from the infected joint capsule. The usually smooth, thin, and tough membrane would be converted to a thick, soft, gelatinous mass. The cartilage it contained would be discolored and ulcerated with detached fragments. All such necrotic tissue must be excised.

Also encased in the joint capsule were the articulating ends of the long bones. If these rounded surfaces were found to be eroded or covered with a dark fleshy growth, they must also be removed with a surgeon's saw. If the bones were smaller, a "rongeur"(gnawing forceps) would do. The diseased joint surfaces would be beveled at the same angle down to healthy bone. A piece of sole leather or a pasteboard card might be used to protect the surrounding soft tissue. It was fortunate that the ailing bone rarely penetrated beyond the epiphysis, those articulating surfaces responsible for the bone's lengthwise growth.

It was hard to believe that the excised joint could still have a degree of flexibility instead of firm bony union. _Syme's Surgery_ of 1857 assured the reader that if rigid splints were not used (as in the Butcher's Box illustration below), "the union is established by means of a tough, flexible, ligamentous-like substance that permits the bones to be used with more or less freedom, according to the exercise which they are made to undergo during the process of healing."

Any small bleeders were tied and the skin closed with widely interrupted sutures to permit postoperative drainage. A lint compress would be changed twice a day, and, finally, sticking plaster tapes would be used to close any skin gaps.

BONE RESECTION

A long bone wounded by a bullet or bayonet and perhaps fragmented could be counted upon to create an extending inflammation. The usual amputation could halt its spread, or resection could be given a try. A swollen enlargement of the shaft with softening, ulceration, and a purulent discharge or a splintered fracture could be excised with a chain handsaw. One end of the flexible chain was attached to a thread and curved needle. Once the needle had passed under the bone to be cut, the threaded chain could be brought up and attached to its handle. With the soft tissues guarded by a thin metal strip, the flexible chain saw handles were raised up and down to begin the sawing. Two cuts were made to free the diseased section. The shortened extremity would be placed in rigid splints for healing. If the excision involved a section of a leg long bone, an elevated shoe was a much happier solution than wearing a peg leg.

"BUTCHER'S SAW" FOR EXCISIONS AND NOT RECOMMENDED FOR AMPUTATIONS

CURVED RONGEUR

LISTON'S BONE FORCEPS

FERGUSSON'S LION FORCEPS FOR HOLDING BONES

GOUGE FOR REMOVING DEAD BONE SECTIONS

"BUTCHER'S BOX" AFTER KNEE EXCISION

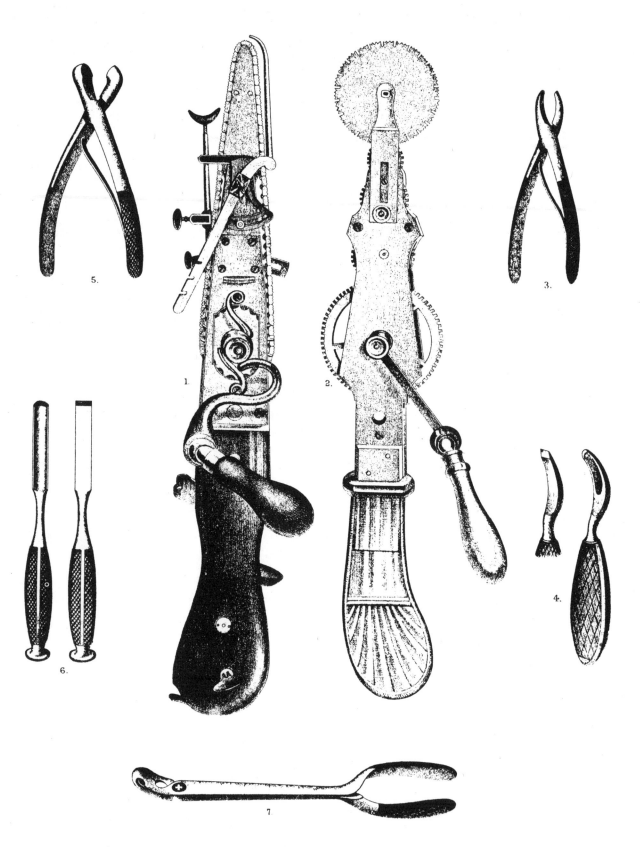

1. Heine's Osteotome.
2. Scie á Móllet.
3.5. Gnawing bone forceps.

PLATE XLI. INSTRUMENTS FOR RESECTION.

4. Legouest's curved gouge and chisel.
6. Gouge and chisel, U.S.A. pattern.
7. Nélaton's bone forceps.

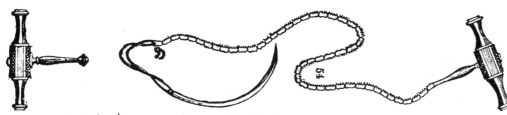

But it wasn't all that simple. Excisions carried out in the rough and tumble of war could have none of the niceties of a clean and well-equipped civilian hospital with a competent surgeon behind the scalpel. A Manual of Military Surgery, Confederate States Army of 1863, put it this way:

"Without undertaking to decide, we simply ask, if, in moving armies upon such a continent as this, it be not better, in order to save life, to amputate immediately upon the field, rather than leave the patient the chance of having his limb preserved by the removal to a distant hospital? When we reflect that the present is a war of immense distances, over huge mountains and along rugged roads, and in which transportation of even the best character is attended with pain, annoyance, sleeplessness, hunger and thirst to the wounded soldier, should not such an operation as will most probably save life, rather than one which preserving limb for a few days, and finally ending in death from either pyaemia, erysipelas or nervous exhaustion be performed?

"In cases hereinafter to be reported, we will find that amputation is best suited to transportation, and resection to absolute rest and care.

"The reasons, as just inferred for this last remark, are based upon the facts that—

1. Resections are of slow performance.
2. They should be well rested after operation.
3. Careful attendance and watchfulness should be for a long time kept over them.
4. Transportation destroys proper adjustment.
5. Long and continued jolting creates suppuration.
6. This, added to want of nervous and muscular power, creates that state of constitution that finally,
7. Ends in death by the causes above enumerated."

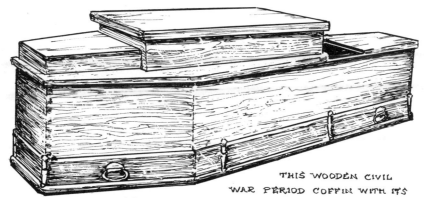

THIS WOODEN CIVIL WAR PERIOD COFFIN WITH ITS ICEBOX ATOP COULD CARRY A SOLDIER'S BODY HOMEWARD FOR A FINAL VIEWING AND BURIAL.
NATIONAL MUSEUM OF CIVIL WAR MEDICINE, FREDERICK, MARYLAND

It was clear that resections were in the province of the general hospitals. To summarize the bottom line on how well the resection technique could compete with the usual amputation, we refer to <u>The War of the Rebellion</u> Part III, Vol. II. "The many favorable results [of resection] leave beyond doubt the wisdom of the course. Still, there was a wide difference of opinion on this point, particularly between field surgeons and those in charge of general hospitals at the rear ~ a difference that can be reconciled by viewing the subject from the standpoint of each."

Further: "Toward the latter part of the war the most thoughtful surgeon found it necessary to exercise careful discrimination in the selection of cases for excision, and to refuse to operate in many instances in which, early in the contest, this operation would have been favored." The promise of this relatively new surgical technique would be advanced once the germ theory became fact and aseptic operations became the rule rather than the exception.

And amputations would be phased out, much to the relief of both surgeons and patients.

THIS REVOLUTIONARY WAR CRUTCH
WAS LITTLE CHANGED DURING THE CIVIL WAR.

SKULL FRACTURE EXCISIONS

There were other bony excisions that required more specialized instruments than the usual surgeon's saw and the flexible chain handsaw. Depressed fractures of the skull presented just that sort of challenge. A simple fracture might give a headache to the patient but none to the surgeon, for such undisplaced cracks healed by themselves. But when detached pieces of the brain's bony helmet caused underlying pressure and perhaps further damage from a growing hematoma, a timely surgical response at the field or the general hospital was in order.

The soldier's head would be shaved and an incision made over the scalp injury. Any detached fractured bony splinters might be removed with forceps without much effort. But when a depressed piece of the bony plate was unyielding in its former site or wedged under fragments, there was no room to pry up the offender. The fracture line must be bored to permit some sort of leverage. This was the work for a T-shaped trephine or perhaps its earlier and less used relative, the trepan that functioned as a brace and bit.

The business end of the trephine was a drum-shaped cutting head with spiral blades that ended in a circle of teeth. The older shape was that of a cylinder, and it cut a disc of bone out of the skull so easily that there was danger of damaging the brain tissue and its protective membrane, the dura mater. Far safer was the newer cutting head with a truncated cone shape that acted as a brake against its cranial walls. But before the trephining began, a perforator pin was lowered

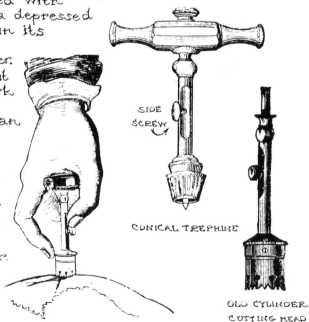

TREPAN WITH SCALP INCISION FLAPS

SIDE SCREW

CONICAL TREPHINE

OLD CYLINDER CUTTING HEAD

THE CYLINDRICAL TREPHINE IN ACTION

from the shaft to just slightly below the circle of teeth and locked with its side screw.

SKULL DISCS WERE TREPHINED TO ALLOW A DEPRESSED FRACTURE PIECE TO BE PRIED UP WITH THE ELEVATOR.

EXAMPLES OF HEY'S SAWS

THE HEY'S SAWS TRIMMED OBSTRUCTING FRACTURE EDGES BEFORE PRYING UP THE LOOSE BONE.

AN ELEVATOR LEVERED AGAINST FIRM BONE TO RAISE A FREED DEPRESSED FRACTURE.

ELEVATOR

THE DOME-SHAPED LENTICULAR TIP PROTECTED THE BRAIN TISSUE WHILE THE BLADE ABOVE CUT AWAY ANY REMAINING RIM OF BONE LEFT BY THE TREPHINE.

With the perforator pin centered over the fracture line and the trephine held perpendicular to the skull, the turning of the handles rotated the cutting head. Once a circular groove of even depth was made, the perforator pin could be retracted and locked well up in the shaft. The trephining was stopped short of reaching the brain membrane with the bone disc not quite detached.

An elevator levered the disc free, leaving a roughened inner rim to the cut hole. This was then smoothed after inserting the lenticular knife between it and the dura mater.

The exposed dura mater membrane should show no evidence of bulging from subdural bleeding that might need incising and draining. If not the trephine hole could be covered with a lead plate or a plug of wax. Any attached and jagged pieces of bone should be trimmed with bone nippers ("rongeur") or with a Hey's saw. If a hematoma was draining, only a piece of linen with perforations followed by lint and compresses would do for bandaging. If no discharge was present, the flaps of the skin incision could be closed with adhesive plaster.

For gunshots alone, the Union Army surgeons trephined 196 soldiers: 110, or 56 percent died, and, of this number, 46 of the trephined deaths were primary operations at the field hospitals. Of the remainder in the general hospitals, 99 of the deaths were intermediary, and 17 were secondary. As for the more fortunate 86 soldiers who survived, nature gradually sealed over the trephined hole with a tough fibroid tissue. But all in all many Civil War surgeons were questioning the value of the trephine and the high mortality rate that accompanied it (see Sidelight 13).

numbers don't add up!

AIRBORNE PESTS

The updated military general hospital must have seemed like a mini-paradise to its recuperating casualties after their battlefield and field hospital ordeals. Even so, purulent drainage from multiple wounds puckered the nose despite the state-of-the-art ventilation systems and efforts to change dressings frequently. These by-products of wound contamination and septic surgery invited clouds of houseflies, black flies, no-see-ums, mosquitoes, horseflies, and other such winged miseries through unscreened windows. The insects would also be tracking smells from any delayed or inadequate garbage or sewage disposal. And some of those flies would leave behind a new generation of their larva.

Letters containing stories of maggots infesting battlefield wounds horrified many of the folks back home. Typical breeding grounds were where the casualties lay for lengthy periods during protracted battles such as the Wilderness and Spottsylvania. Difficult ambulance retrieval and too few attendants at the general hospital when they finally arrived compounded the problem. Even under several layers of muslin bandaging, the maggots~ probably either deposited by the bluebottle flies or houseflies~ were in plenty.

H.S. Schell, Assistant Surgeon, U.S.A., wrote this note in June 1862 after the Peninsular Campaign's Gaines' Mill battle:

"But while food was scarce maggots were abundant crowding and rolling over every wound, and searching beneath the dressings to fasten upon every excoriation. Oil of turpentine and infusion of tobacco and the flowers of elderberry were tried, for the purpose of getting rid of this pest; but the most effectual means was found to be dressing forceps; and to keep the wound clean, it required to be examined every two or three hours. A solution of camphor in oil is an excellent remedy, if applied directly to the bodies of the intruders, the secretions of the wound having previously been removed by a piece of sponge. It seems to me that the maggot actually does damage in a wound; although not by attacking the living tissues, but only by the annoyance created by the continual sensation of crawling and irritation which it occasions, and of which the patient often complains bitterly. In certain states of the system, the nervous excitement or irritability thus engendered must react injuriously upon the parts."

As it turned out, Confederate doctors attending prisoners in Chattanooga in 1863 discovered the maggot problem WASN'T much of a problem. Their bandaging and disinfectants had run out and wounds could no longer be dressed. Maggots had free reign. To the surgeons' surprise, the maggots consumed only the dead and diseased tissue, leaving a clean and viable wound surface behind.

THE DUTY ROSTER

Each Union general hospital was the responsibility of its surgeon in charge. Besides their regular and volunteer medical ward officer staff, many doctors served under contract for duty with forces in

THE HOSPITAL WARD
VENTILATION SYSTEM COMBATTED NOXIOUS AIR ("MAL-ARIA")

the field or in the general hospitals. These private physicians without commissions were called acting assistant surgeons. They were numerous and included many eminent surgeons and physicians. Also assigned to ward duty in the general hospital were medical students serving as wound dressers, managing the dispensary and serving as general assistants.

Hospital stewards * were noncommissioned officers with

* THE CADUCEUS WAS FIRST WORN BY HOSPITAL STEWARDS IN 1851 AS A SLEEVE EMBLEM. EMBROIDERED IN GREEN. THEY WERE THE FORERUNNERS OF THE MEDICAL NONCOMMISSIONED OFFICERS OF TODAY. A LITTLE LATER IT SERVED AS A METALLIC CAP INSIGNIA FOR THE STEWARDS. THE CADUCEUS HAS BEEN WORN BY MEMBERS OF THE MEDICAL CORPS SINCE 1902 WITH A SUPER-IMPOSED "D" FOR DENTAL, "V" FOR VETERINARY, "A" FOR ADMINISTRATIVE, "S" FOR SANITARY OFFICERS, AND "N" FOR NURSES.

different responsibilities. One, with some pharmaceutical background would have charge of the dispensary and medical property. Another would be the quartermaster-sergeant who issued and recorded such supplies as clothing and blankets. A steward would also be in charge of subsistence, drawing rations and issuing such to the kitchens. Sometimes a steward would act as chief wardmaster over the wards.

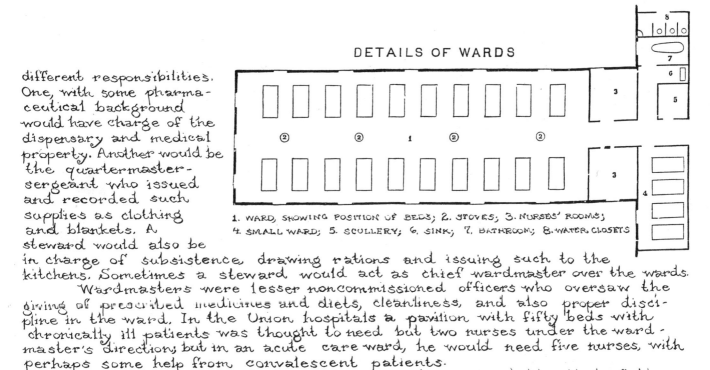

DETAILS OF WARDS

1. WARD, SHOWING POSITION OF BEDS; 2. STOVES; 3. NURSES' ROOMS; 4. SMALL WARD; 5. SCULLERY; 6. SINK; 7. BATHROOM; 8. WATER CLOSETS

Wardmasters were lesser noncommissioned officers who oversaw the giving of prescribed medicines and diets, cleanliness, and also proper discipline in the ward. In the Union hospitals a pavilion with fifty beds with chronically ill patients was thought to need but two nurses under the ward-master's direction; but in an acute care ward, he would need five nurses, with perhaps some help from convalescent patients.

The Confederate hospital command was much like that of the Union's — with several exceptions. Both Northern and Southern general hospitals pressed convalescing soldiers into service for nursing duties initially, but female nursing and the Veteran Reserve Corps would be important Union hospital innovations ahead.

ARMY NURSING

Maggots, lice, wound dressings, and washing patients, scrubbing ward floors, emptying bedpans, and a variety of other onerous chores were the lot of army hospital ward attendants. Untrained and unenthusiastic, they were detailed to such duty while recuperating from illness or injury, having a physical handicap, or just not particularly good soldier material. It was drudgery akin to peeling a mountain of potatoes for the daily mess. General hospital nursing was not one of medicine's great adventures as far as those makeshift nurses were concerned.

FEMALE NURSES

There remained another possibility: trained, efficient, and caring female army nurses. Perhaps the women who labored in pre-Civil War civilian hospitals and local almshouses were considered on a lower rung of the social ladder. No doubt the average mother, wife, and homemaker would agree with Florence Nightingale when she remarked that such hospital helpers "were generally those who were too old, too weak, too drunken, too dirty, too stolid, or too bad to do anything else." Many would question the propriety of decent female nurses cast among sick and wounded soldiers where the long exhausting hours might be intermixed with raging hormones. Still Miss Nightingale's successes with her trained nursing staff of women in the Crimean War deserved a second look in America with a civil war close at hand.

Petite Dorothea Lynde Dix had already made her mark as a dedicated reformer for the mentally ill. She had taken Nurse Nightingale's lessons to heart and set out for Washington as the first wave of volunteers was hurrying to the defense of the Capital. Although Miss Dix was but 5 feet tall, she carried with her more than enough determination to make up for first impressions when she met with acting Surgeon General Wood. When she left his office, she had been given the title of "superintendent of female nurses for the Union Army." Congress followed through by authorizing the employment of female nurses in the army's general hospitals.

Miss Dix answered the concerns over the intermixing of men and women with her own rigid requirements for prospective nurses. No candidate need apply if she was not thirty years of age or older. She should have plain features that wouldn't turn a man's head and wear only simple dresses unencumbered with bustles. She must at all times exhibit decorum while on her rounds. Limited training would be given before assignment, and the pay would be 40 cents a day plus rations.

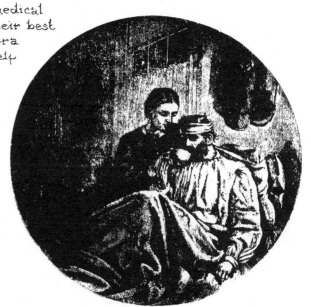

DOROTHEA DIX

Superintendent Dix's rules and regulations seemed an obstacle course for patriotic women who wished to become nurses. One recruit called her "a self-sealing can of horror tied up in red tape." More than that she lacked the administrative and organizational skills necessary for so large an undertaking. Unable to delegate authority, she became exhausted inspecting the hospitals on her own. Finally the Medical Department took control of all nursing appointments and then the supervision of the nurses after joining the army. Although Miss Dix had become little more than a figurehead, she had introduced female nursing into the male world of American warfare.

Although the women's liberation movement was many years in the future, "pretty young things" were gradually being admitted to nursing because of competence and not appearance. Over 3,200 female nurses had joined the Union's war effort when peace was finally declared. Still prejudice among the hospital doctors limited their usefulness. The Medical and Surgical History of the Rebellion put it this way:

"According to the testimony of all the medical officers who have referred to this point their best service was rendered in connection with extra diets, the linen-room and laundry. Male help was preferred in the wards, save in special cases of prostration and suffering where particular care was needful in the administration of dietetic or remedial agents. Sometimes where no female aid was employed, females and societies volunteered their services in superintending the extra diets and taking charge of the contribution room."

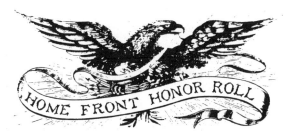

HOME FRONT HONOR ROLL

Southern tradition seemed dead set against its ladies taking any part in the life-and-death struggle for secession. But not everyone kept to the isolation of the home, hearth, and children mindset. When the Union offensives tightened around the South later in the war, many wives and sweethearts provided rest stops for their battlefield casualties. Unfortunately most of their contributions have gone unrecorded.

Sally L. Tompkins was appalled by the lack of decent general hospital facilities for the Rebel troops after the First Battle of Bull Run. She not only organized and operated the Robertson Hospital in Richmond, she used her own savings for it as well. It was one of the many independent hospitals established without government help, but in time all were taken over by the military with an officer placed in charge of each. Miss Tompkins wasn't about to be sidelined; she appealed directly to President Jefferson Davis. Her good works were already known, and the Confederate president commissioned her with the rank of captain. She could then continue her work at Robertson Hospital ~ naming it the Tompkins Hospital would seem to have been more appropriate ~ as the one and only Rebel woman officer in the Civil War.

It was a group of public-spirited women who persuaded the Confederate Congress in 1862 to begin hiring those of their gender for general hospital duty. As the new law read, women were to be employed as hospital matrons to superintend "the entire domestic economy of the hospital, to take charge of such delicacies as may be provided for the sick, to apportion them out as desired, to see that the food or diet is properly prepared, and all such other duties as may be necessary." Assistant matrons were given the responsibility for the laundry, the clothing of the sick, and the hospital bedding." (C.S. Statutes 1 Cong., 2 Sess., chapter 17, 1862).

Hospital housekeeping was a far cry from the actual hands-on "nursing" required of recuperating soldiers. But Kate Cumming (1828-1909) was bound she'd follow Florence Nightingale's example dispite her family's admonition that "nursing soldiers was no work for a refined lady." She joined some forty other untrained women from Mobile. They arrived in northern Mississippi just in time to be engulfed by a flood of the wounded from the Shiloh battlefield.

NURSE KATE CUMMING

Most of Kate's companions, unable to cope with so great a scale of human destruction, returned home. For the next three years she worked in Confederate general hospitals as a matron ~ a job made doubly difficult because of the prejudices of that time. As she wrote in her diary "[A] lady's respectability must be at a low ebb when it can be endangered by going into a hospital."

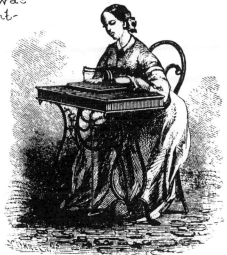

HOME FRONT CONTRIBUTIONS

And therein lies her most important contribution to history ~ her down-to-earth daily record of life in the Confederate hospitals. In 1866 she returned to Mobile and had the first-hand accounts published as <u>A Journal of Hospital Life in the Confederate Army of Tennessee</u>. The book was reprinted in 1959 at Birmingham as <u>Kate: The Journal of a Confederate Nurse</u>.

There were many ways that women contributed to the health and welfare of their Union fighting men. The following thumbnail sketches point out a few of the determined and spirited women who went the extra mile for their country.

The mention of Louisa May Alcott (1832-1888) brings to mind such classic books as <u>Little Women</u>, <u>Little Men</u>, <u>Under the Lilacs</u>, and <u>Eight Cousins</u>. Yet few readers today know of her first published <u>Hospital Sketches</u> in 1863 and its impact on the Union's Civil War effort. Before Sumpter, her home town of Concord, Massachusetts, and the rest of New England were solidly behind the preservation of the <u>united</u> states. Her family boarded the daughters of John Brown, the anti-slavery zealot who gave his life at Harper's Ferry. When war was declared, Louisa May exchanged her Boston schoolmarm career for army nursing. Although her efforts were cut short by a bout of typhoid fever, her letters home were published in the influential <u>Hospital Sketches</u>. Her impressions of the wounded soldiers at the Union Hospital

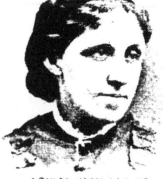

LOUISA MAY ALCOTT

at Georgetown brought a deeper understanding of the sacrifices being made into many a Northern parlor.

Julia Ward Howe (1819-1910) was another author well known for her writings, lectures, and social reforms. But she is best remembered for the November of 1861 when she was caught in a Washington traffic jam. To pass the time, she began singing the soldiers' song "John Brown's Body." Troops passing by her open carriage picked up the tune, and one of her party suggested that she write more stirring lyrics to the old hymn's melody. Dawn the following day found Mrs. Howe busy composing

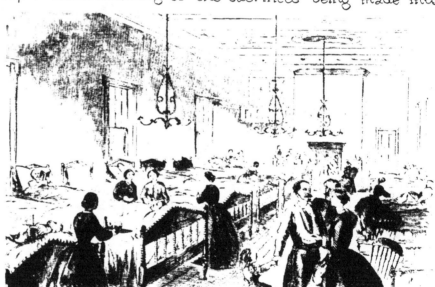

THE UNITED STATES HOSPITAL AT GEORGETOWN, FORMERLY THE UNION HOTEL, WHERE LOUISA MAY ALCOTT SERVED AS A NURSE IN 1862.

the words to "The Battle Hymn of the Republic." It soon became the inspiration of the Union troops as they marched into battle, and it is said that President Lincoln wept upon hearing it sung.

When Kady Brownell (1842-19?) said her marriage vows, she had no idea that she'd soon be in the fury of a battlefield. But when war was declared, her new husband promptly volunteered in the First Rhode Island Infantry. Kady had no intention of being left behind. Her determination won the duty of color bearer in his company of sharpshooters. Mrs. Brownell

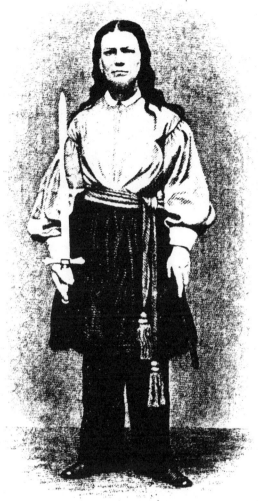

KADY BROWNELL

carried her sergeant's sword and became a deadly shot with a rifle. There was no time, however, for either weapon to be used when the Union line broke into a retreat at Bull Run. Instead she held her flag as a rallying point for the company. She cheated death when the soldier next to her was killed by a cannonball.

In a later battle at Newbern during the Peninsula Campaign, she was twice ordered not to carry the regimental colors during a charge on the Rebel lines. Some accounts say that she was wounded in action there as was her husband. We do know that his fractured thigh bone brought his soldiering career to an end. Kady Brownell nursed her husband in the hospital for some eighteen months until the couple could be discharged. She returned home with her prized sword, the flag she'd carried, and a good many memories.

Mary Morris Husband (dates unknown) brought a touch of home to the Union Army hospitals. Her travels throughout the eastern theater of war began in the summer of 1862 aboard a transport bound for the Peninsula Campaign wounded. After three such voyages Mrs. Husband began matron duty in the field and general hospitals until the end of the rebellion. She seemed everywhere: Washington, Alexandria, Baltimore, Antietam, Brandy Station, Fredericksburg, Chancellorsville, Battle of the Wilderness, and Richmond. Yet there was always time for recuperating soldiers to stop by her tent for books, games, writing paper, or a chat. She was known for her great apron with ample pockets that held apples, newspapers, stockings, a Testament, handkerchiefs, and other such gifts. She also gave of herself, such as the time she didn't hesitate going to the secretary of war or the president himself when she learned of extenuating circumstances that might save the life of a soldier condemned to death.

MARY MORRIS HUSBAND

The common soldiers' spirited protector on the western front was Mary Ann Byckerdyke (1817-1901). The middle-aged widow volunteered to work with the Western Sanitation Commission in Cairo with another independent thinker, Mary Jane Safford. Known to soldiers and officers alike as "Mother," Mrs. Byckerdyke stood for no nonsense in her calling. One example told around the campfires took place after the Fort Donelson battle just over the Kentucky border. She discovered that a surgeon had diverted jellies, wines, and other Commission supplies for the wounded to his own table. Mother Byckerdyke stormed the rascal's tent, snatched up the goods, and hurried straightaway to General Grant. Within twenty-four hours the surgeon was under arrest.

"Mother" Byckerdyke was soon on duty at the Vicksburg siege and then she was off to the battles of Missionary Ridge and Lookout Mountain that overlooked Chattanooga. She was the Sanitary Commission's guarantee that all its provisions would reach the sick and wounded. They could count on a taste from home such as fresh-baked bread, thick hot soup, tea and coffee, and perhaps boiled mutton. When a supply officer formally requested that this purposeful woman be removed from the hospital as an "improper influence" the general asked who she was. "A Mrs. Byckerdyke," replied the major. "Oh well," said the general, "she outranks me; you must apply to President Lincoln."

"MOTHER" MARY ANN BYCKERDYKE

Mary Jane Safford (1834-1891), though described as "very frail" and "petite as a girl of twelve summers," was driven to do everything she could for the battlefield casualties. At strategic Cairo, Kentucky, where the Ohio joined the Mississippi River, she skirted the opposition of camp officers and surgeons, making daily rounds with donated newspapers, games and letter-writing materials for the sick and wounded. The Western Sanitary Commission authorized her to draw on other spirit-boosters to be given to the patients. She worked with "Mother" Byckerdyke and made five voyages with her on the Sanitary Commission's transport ship "City of Memphis." When under fire while treating the Belmont battlefield wounded, she tied her white handkerchief to a stick so as not to have her work interrupted. The soldiers

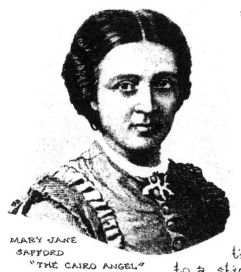

MARY JANE
SAFFORD
"THE CAIRO ANGEL"

dubbed her "the Cairo Angel."

Miss Safford's enthusiasm for helping the ill carried her to a medical degree in 1867. She practiced in Boston, lectured at her medical school, and was active in many reform movements. One such time she called her old friend Mrs. Byckerdyke to come to New York to help clean up the slums. After a four year stint, Dr. Safford raised funds to help Mother Byckerdyke with relief work she was doing among the settlers in Iowa.

Belle Reynolds (1840-19?) had been married just a year to the day when word came of the Fort Sumpter attack. She refused to remain at home when her husband promptly

BELLE REYNOLDS

enlisted as a lieutenant in the Seventeenth Illinois Regiment. She became the nurse in camp and on campaign, and she became so interested in the practice of medicine that she apprenticed for her M.D. degree in 1864 when her husband's tour of duty was over. During her years of practice Dr. Reynolds represented Clara Barton in the Red Cross Service, taking her as far from home as the Philippines.

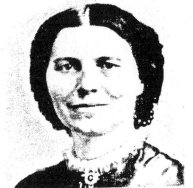

CLARA BARTON
"ANGEL OF THE BATTLEFIELD"

Clara Barton (1821-1912) began her nursing career in September 1862, just in time for the fury at the Antietam battlefield. She made a timely arrival with a wagonload of badly needed Sanitary Commission medical supplies. Union surgeons had been using corn husks for bandaging. Bringing medicines and nursing the wounded on the battlefields won her the title "Angel of the Battlefield." In 1864 she was appointed superintendent of nurses for the Army of the James [River].

When the war ended, Miss Barton formed a bureau to search out those servicemen who were missing in action. At the Andersonville Prison in Georgia she and her party were able to mark more than 12,000 graves that otherwise would have remained unknown.

In 1869 she served as a nurse during the Franco-Prussian War. While there she came to appreciate the work of the International Red Cross in Europe. She convinced the United States government that the Geneva Treaty should be ratified. It was not surprising that Miss Barton became the first president of the American Red Cross.

Elizabeth Blackwell (1821-1910) overcame almost impossible hurdles to become America's first woman medical doctor. The Blackwell family emigrated from England in 1832 after losing the family fortune. After settling in Ohio the nine children were left penniless when their father died. Elizabeth taught school in Cincinnati while pursuing her dream of becoming a doctor. It seemed that the goal would remain a dream, for her admission applications to the leading medical schools were rejected because of her sex. Persistance did win out and she was finally accepted by Geneva Medical School in New York State.

Dr. Blackwell graduated with the highest honors in 1849 and continued her internship in Paris ~ where she lost the sight in one eye from an infection ~ and in London. Back in New York, Blackwell organized the New York Infirmary for Women and Children. When war was declared, she formed the Women's Central Association of Relief, which played a prominent role in establishing the United States Sanitary Commission. She and her sister,

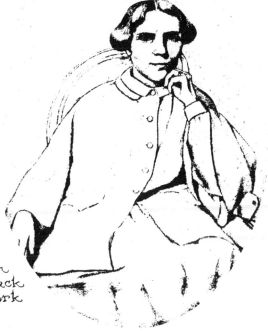

ELIZABETH BLACKWELL IN HER THIRTIES
WEARING HER "DOCTORIAL SACK" IN LONDON

who had earned her own M.D. degree in 1854, helped with the selection and training of the Union Army nurses. Later, in 1873, Elizabeth Blackwell helped in the organization of the first training school for nurses in the United States.

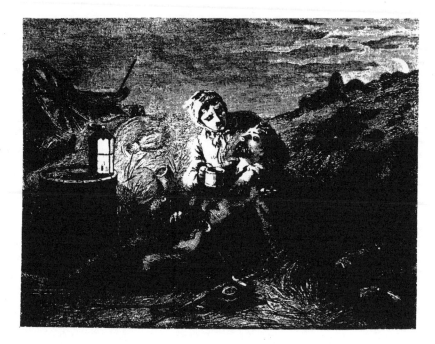

"MOTHER."
MARY ANN BYCKERDYKE
CARING FOR THE WOUNDED
ON THE BATTLEFIELD
AT MIDNIGHT

MALE NURSES

Except for the modest introduction of female nurses in the Union general hospitals, males dominated the nursing duties in the North and exclusively so in the South. As mentioned earlier, most were convalescing soldiers who had neither the interest nor the inclination for ward labor. The alternatives of guard duty and working as a mess hall orderly or clerk were also second best to the excitement and adventure of marching off on campaign. In the Confederate hospitals, there were also free blacks or slaves who could fill in as cooks, waiters, laundresses, wagoneers, carpenters, and on general pick-and-shovel duty.

Such was the state of affairs before the Union's new Surgeon General William Hammond entered the picture. He aimed his innovative reforms at the make-do nursing tradition that would remain unchanged in Rebel country. Congress was quick to approve of his new Army Hospital Corps blueprint. Every army nurse candidate must be physically fit, intelligent, honest, and reliable. Each would be responsible for the hospital's supplies, receiving and distributing rations to the patients and seeing that his patients were well cared for and each ward kept clean and uncluttered. He would enter his nursing duties with the rating of sergeant, wear a special Hospital Corps uniform, and must be under the direct control of the United States Medical Department. This approach to a professionalism in patient care served as a blueprint in the days to come.

There was still a place for the recovering sick and wounded in the hospital setting. The Union Invalid Corps was more a position of honor than busy work. On occasion those near recovery might still be pressed into ward service, but the Corps emphasized its military training with policing, maintaining order, and standing guard duty (see Sidelight 14).

DISEASE CONCEPTS

To summarize what we have discussed thus far, disease prevention was really a Civil War soldier's only hope of avoiding a death-dealing illness (see Sidelight 15). The guidelines had long been emphasized by the

Sanitation Commission: a decent quality and quantity of food, clothing, shelter, and better personal hygiene and camp sanitation. Holding to such standards became increasingly difficult in the last years of the war for the beleaguered Confederate troops. A Yankee bullet posed considerably less danger than the onset of the inflammation symptoms of heat, redness, swelling, and pain. It has been estimated that for every battlefield death, the South lost three times that number of young men to disease. The ratio was a bit better for the Union troops, which had two deaths for the fighting to five who died from illness (see Sidelight 13).

Unfortunately, the theory-based medicines used by physicians were all but useless ~ even harmful at times. The dictates of medical dogma had smothered the theory that unseen invaders might be the villains behind most illnesses. Actually, all those minute round dots and rods had been seen under the microscope. Their presence had been interpreted as part of the body's healing process, along with the abundance of white blood cells. Those "laudable" pus cells were in the process of engulfing the bacteria and were not, as believed, a positive sign that they would win the battle.

Even if the germ theory had been proven before the Civil War, physicians would have been slow accepting such a new and outlandish idea. Dealing in human lives has always made the profession a cautious lot. And so the old cookbook treatments continued as usual for the inflammation diseases. Any soldiers not severely ill would be given medication at their own regimental hospital. Those with more life-threatening or prolonged sicknesses would be sent along to the general hospital in that area.

BAKER'S COMPOUND MICROSCOPE- ENGLISH, c1860

All maladies were classified under the headings of MIASMATIC, NONMIASMATIC ORIGIN, and a catchall of UNCLASSIFIED DISEASES.

MIASMATIC DISEASES

Miasma was the poisonous atmosphere believed to have risen from swamps and putrid matter to cause disease. These airborne miseries were divided into those causing Intermittent, Continued, and Eruptive Fevers. All such miasmatic treatments would attempt to rid the body of its infectious poisons. Such was the goal of the fresh-air ventilation in the pavilion hospitals. A dose of cathartics would first be given to flush out the intestines and then diaphoretics to perspire the toxins away. General symptomatic therapy would then follow as noted on pages 3 to 5. If the fever disease happened to be eruptive, special attention might be given to the skin lesions. Except for a rare medicine such as quinine that really worked, diseases would receive cookbook therapy.

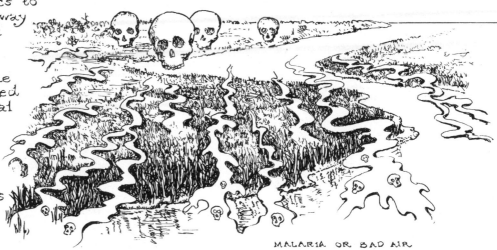

MALARIA OR BAD AIR

INTERMITTENT (PAROXYSMAL) FEVERS ~ These

fevers were otherwise known as malaria (mal-area or bad air). Swamp origins made sense, although no one understood that the anopheles mosquito carried the malarial parasites. These parasites invaded the victim's red blood cells to bring on a shaking chill and then profuse sweating. The intermittent symptoms were caused by the parasites developing in the red blood cells at intervals of as short as a week to as long as many years before rupturing the cell wall and repeating the cyclic symptoms.

Quinine, also called Peruvian Bark because of its South American cinchona bark derivation, was a clear and bitter liquid. It was one of the very few medicines that was specific for a cure in those days. When a Northern port blockade interrupted the Southern quinine supply, turpentine was applied externally as an alternative therapy for malarial symptoms. Confederate Surgeon General Moore found the turpentine treatment "amply sufficient to interrupt the morbific chain of successive paroxysms one application only being required in the majority of cases." Other substitutes included a tonic brewed from the bark of the dogwood, poplar, and willow trees dissolved in whiskey.

CONTINUED FEVERS ~ These

fevers were known to the soldiers as "Camp Fevers" or "Crowd-poisonings" with good reason. When masses of troops were packed into the confines of a campground, the Continued Fevers raced through the ranks. It was believed that bad air, poor ventilation, or organic matter fermenting in the soil were causing the ongoing temperatures. Typhoid was one such disease that was indeed caused by Salmonella bacteria. Contaminated water supplies or flies carrying feces to food gave weight to the basic objective of the United States Sanitary Commission's Olmsted: "prevention rather than cure." Without the safeguards of clean water, personal cleanliness and proper privies, the Confederate soldier had twice the risk of becoming a typhoid patient.

Those who ingested the germs would soon advertise that fact with a gradually rising temperature, sometimes

CATALOGUE

Utensils, Surgical Instruments, etc.

BULLOCK & CRENSHAW, PHILADELPHIA. 1857.

SADDLE-BAGS, for Physicians:—

The Bags here described are made of fine white Leather. The sides worn next to the horse are without seam. A flap of Patent Leather covers the tops of the Bags, and protects them from the weather. The edges of the flaps are neatly trimmed with red. The Bottles contained in all of them, are glass-stoppered.

Fig. 75.

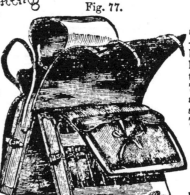

serves for carrying Instruments, Packages, &c., (Fig. 75,)

The bottles in this Bag are contained in drawers, which slide in at the ends of the bag, and are fastened by a strap passing through an eye in the drawer—the eyes serve as handles, by which the drawers are drawn out. The drawers containing the medicines, can be removed without taking the bags from the horse. A space above the drawers

Bags containing 24 vials,	.	11 00
" " 20 "	.	10 00
" " 16 "	.	9 00

Fig. 76.

The bottles are at the bottom of the bag —(as shown in the section)—a tray is placed above the bottles for carrying Instruments, &c, The tray must be removed to gain access to the bottles, (Fig 76.)

Bags containing 24 vials,	$11 00
Bags containing 20 vials,	10 00
Bags containing 16 vials,	9 00

Fig. 77.

Flat Bags—(as shown in the figure) —a row of small bottles above the larger ones, are intended for Powders. The inside flap has a pocket in it for Instruments, &c., (Fig. 77.)

Bags containing 32 vials,	12 00
Bags containing 28 vials,	11 00

The above Bags, made entirely of Patent Leather; will be furnished at $3 additional. A sheet of Labels will be furnished with the Bags.

rose-colored skin spots, an enlarged spleen, and, later, diarrhea, delirium, stupor, and perhaps death. As for treatment, you may remember Dr. Brown's Indirect Inflammation theory on pages 3 to 5: the symptomatic treatments he recommended in typhoid fever cases were cathartics or mild purgatives and diaphoretics, localized bleeding, narcotics, and counterirritants. If the patient should lapse into delerium or coma despite these heroic efforts, a paste of Spanish Fly blisters could be applied over the patient's shaved scalp.

Typhus certainly qualified as a "crowd poisoning" continued fever. The body louse carried rickettsia ~ minute round bodies halfway between viruses and bacteria ~ to their unwilling soldier hosts. Although too tiny to be seen by the ordinary microscope, the resulting signs and symptoms were clear enough. Chills, then fever with a scattering of reddish spots over the abdomen were the rickettsia's calling cards during the first twenty-four hours. Restlessness followed, then convulsions, coma, and perhaps death.

The body louse's breeding grounds developed wherever close-quartered troops lived in unsanitary conditions. The Union's sanitary report in December 1861 bristled with exasperation following a general camp inspection. The volunteer regimental officers rarely enforced the general order for clean feet, neck, and heads and noted "the slovenly, slipshod appearance of the clothing and accouterments, their filthy skins, uncombed hair, and matted beards." Unwashed clothing and lack of bathing water seemed a way of life in the confusion of the early war months. The Commission continued its concentrated efforts to educate the rank and file of the Union Army.

<u>The Life of Johnny Reb</u> tells of an Alabama soldier writing home in 1863 that "there is not a man in the army, officer or private that doesn't have from a battalion to a Brigade of Body lice on him." When the wife of another Rebel soldier from the same state suggested visiting camp with their two children, he wrote back "if you was here the Boddy lice would eat up Booth of the children in one knight in spite of all we doo; you don't hav any idea what sort of animal they are." And another Confederate was heard complaining that "I get vexed at them and commence killing them, but as I believe forty come to every one's funeral, I have given it up as a bad job." It was said that Rebel soldiers claimed the body louse was such a part of their army that the big "graybacks" wore the letters C.S. for Confederate States.

THE HOUSEFLY

ADULT

EGGS

LARVA

PUPA

STAGES IN DEVELOPMENT OF THE HOUSEFLY

THE BODY LOUSE SPORTING A TOUCH OF SOUTHERN HUMOR.

ERUPTIVE FEVERS ~ These fevers exhibited a varied sprinkling of skin eruptions with the rise in temperature. Among the Civil War soldiers, measles seemed to be the most frequent and most incapacitating. One out seven Union recruits in the summer of 1861 were in the regimental hospitals with the disease. It was reported that the rebels were so riddled with the illness that companies, battalions, and whole regiments had to be disbanded for a time and sent home. They received the usual fever medicines and perhaps mild topical applications to the itchy (pruritus) flat to slightly raised (maculopapular) brownish pink lesions.

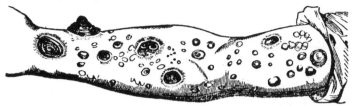
AN ASSORTMENT OF SKIN LESIONS

Smallpox (variola) was a disfiguring, life-threatening disease that could be the lot of any soldier who hadn't had his cowpox vaccination. Sometimes the vaccine itself was just as dangerous, as many Confederate troops discovered before mobilizing for the May 1863 battle of Chancellorville. The vaccine was contaminated with bacteria, and the spreading infections were interpreted by the theories of the day as due to "epidemic atmosphere." As many as 5,000 men were unfit for duty after receiving the germ-laced cowpox. The treatment would be the same as that prescribed for all fevers. The treatment of smallpox skin lesions might start with applications of cool water, a mixture of milk and water, or perhaps a lead-water poultice (acetate of lead in a watery solution) to the developing blisterlike vesicles. These blebs holding clear serum were sometimes lanced and drained to decrease irritation and pitting. When the vesicles became pustules, plasters with mercurial or sulphuric ointment might be used over the face. The masklike plaster was occlusive to prevent the lesions from developing further by contact with noxious air. And yet the blisters erupted as usual.

OPENING A SKIN LESION

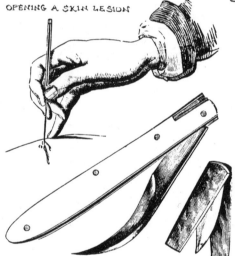

SYME'S ABSCESS LANCET

ABSCESS LANCET

Erysipelas made its sudden appearance with a high fever and a circumscribed reddened, hot, and swollen patch of skin. Because it appeared in the winter months, the cause was believed to be tainted warmth in confined spaces at the expense of fresh air. Actually it was the hemolytic streptococci that caused the rapidly spreading "inflammatory blush" and swelling in the subcutaneous tissue. In addition to the fever medicines, many different topical applications such as tincture of iodine or a sprinkling of rye meal were put on in a futile effort to draw out the poisons. Many a general hospital doctor or nurse likely caught the contageon from lancing surface blisters and abscesses. They, too, would be open to such complications as pneumonia, gangrene, and septicemia that might well lead to coma and death. Isolation to prevent the "dissipation of causative miasmas" was combined with free ventilation of pavilion hospitals, washing or burning of clothes, and smearing the body with oil, fresh lard, or glycerine.

Yellow fever was considered an eruptive fever by virtue of the minute hemorrhagic spots (petechiae) on the skin and a generalized yellow tint with jaundice from extensive liver damage. It was believed that the airborne miasmas from Cuba brought the disease. There was a wisp of truth to the theory, for it was the female Aëdes aegypt (the Greeks were right on target,"Aëdes" means unpleasant, unfriendly) mosquito carrying the yellow fever virus. Heroic systematic treatment would be given, for death was a frequent visitor with this disease when it was epidemic among the troops. Then as now, removing the troops from swampy and low moist areas until frost was a prophylaxis learned from experience. Even today we have no specific treatment for the yellow fever virus, as with most other viral infections.

Other miasmatic diseases less seen in the Civil War ranks were the plague, scarlet fever (scarlatina), glanders, dengue, and milk sickness.

NONMIASMATIC DISEASES

Cold and dampness, not poisonous air, were the causes of many respiratory tract inflammations. Assorted bacteria were the undiscovered culprits. It was thought that cold and dampness could invade one's respiratory tract and cause such diseases as coryza, otherwise known as acute inflammation of the nostrils, tonsillitis, quinsy (now called tonsillar abscess), and diphtheria. The lungs were the farthest away for inhaled moist, cold air, bringing an inflammation called pneumonia. An inflammatory extension could involve the outer linings of the lungs and the inner chest wall with pleurisy. These pleural membranes gave intense sharp, stabbing pains with every deep breath or cough.

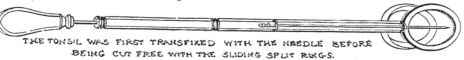

TONSILOTOME

THE TONSIL WAS FIRST TRANSFIXED WITH THE NEEDLE BEFORE BEING CUT FREE WITH THE SLIDING SPLIT RINGS.

Treatment followed the usual fever medications, with a tracheotomy needed for labored respirations. The only indication for bleeding in the general hospitals was excessive breathing difficulties. It was thought, according to Wood's Practice of Medicine, Volume II 1858, that "by diminishing the amount of blood, we relieve the lung of a portion of this duty." On the contrary the remaining healthy lung tissue had to bear twice the workload with a nonfunctioning lung and less oxygen-carrying blood from bleeding.

THE TRACHEOTOMY TUBE WAS INSERTED INTO THE WINDPIPE.

In The Life of Johnny Reb, it was noted that "mustard plasters were popular for chest and bronchial infections. One soldier who dispaired of cure by his doctor sought haven in a private home where, according to his testimony, he 'prety well burnt the pleurasy out of [his] side with pepper and Number six and hot bricks.'" Many Rebs wore flannel bands about their waists to fend off ill effects of exposure to dampness and cold. The Confederates had other homemade remedies up their sleeves. A cold could be cured by drinking as much molasses and water at bedtime as one could hold. Or a pint of tea of roasted or baked apples before sleep would do the trick. And for cough, a teaspoon of vinegar and salt mixture should be taken several times a day.

Rheumatism, also believed to be provoked by the cold and dampness, brought the owner such miseries as joint and muscle pain, tenderness, stiffness, and swelling. More times than not, back pain (lumbago), sore neck (wry neck or torticollis), thorax pain (pleurodynia), and aching shoulders and thighs (charley horse) were caused by strained fibromuscular tissue. The hefty weight of the knapsack and equipment seemed almost

THE RHEUMATIC DODGER
FAKING JOINT PAIN

guaranteed to place a strain on one's musculature. Veteran troops soon learned to leave behind or discard such weighty concerns and carry only the rifle and ammunition along with a change of underclothing wrapped in the blanket roll. Such stripped-down luggage could be slung over the shoulder and the free ends tied together over the opposite hip.

A red, swollen, and painful joint was quite another story. These were ominous signs of acute inflammation that could end in bacterial blood poisoning (septicemia). Multiple painfully inflamed joints could also mean rheumatic fever from a streptococcal infection. The delayed arthritic symptoms would subside and disappear without further problems, but many victims developed a coexisting inflamed heart with destruction of the heart valves. Many a soldier who had rheumatic fever as a youngster would suffer heart failure during the uncompromising duties of a campaign.

Chronic arthritis would be evident in the more senior soldiers in damp cold weather. Most complaints would signal the wear-and-tear joints of osteoarthritis, enlarged and painful through years of use, injury, or low calcium intake. Many advanced cases were discharged from the service~thereby presenting a real problem for the doctor and the army itself. The arthritis diagnosis was based mainly on symptoms and not physical signs, thereby giving the Sunday soldier or malingerer a possible escape from the discomforts, rigors, and dangers of military life.

It might seem strange that scurvy was considered a chronic rheumatic disease. Dr. James Lind, a Scottish naval surgeon, puzzled that sailors on long voyages developed bleeding from spongy gums, failure of wounds to heal, liver-colored skin patches from bleeding subcutaneous capillaries~and aching joints. In 1747 Lind found that lemon and lime juice actually prevented this multiplicity of symptoms, and British tars were thereafter known as limeys. Thanks to his efforts, scurvy was the one and only vitamin deficiency disease known to the Civil War physicians.

The symptoms of scurvy's lack of vitamin C were caused by defective intracellular cementing tissue that allowed leaking of blood throughout the body. The dull aching pains in the extremities were provoked by hemorrhages into the muscles and joints. Preventable, perhaps, but difficult to achieve when citrus fruits, melons, peppers, greens, cabbage, strawberries and potatoes were not in season. Otherwise the winter and early spring diet of salt beef or pork, bean or pea soup, hardtack, and coffee remained the diet mainstays. The United States Army was able to store potatoes in quantity, but few troops bothered to take them along on a march.

Desiccated vegetables, mentioned briefly under the RATIONS heading, seemed like an answer for the Union troops. One of McClellan's Army of the Potomac soldiers, Private Joseph Bellard, gave us his impression of the fare. In his diary under November 27, 1861, he wrote that "the desacated vegetables were all kinds of green stuf pressed into a square cake, and when we wanted any soup a piece of it was broken off and put in the pot, when it would swell out and make a very nice soup." Private Bellard seemed to be in the minority, however, for McClellan's Medical Director Tripler found

AIFHI!

that the soldiers "very generally refused to use the desiccated vegetables." By April 1862, scurvy was a definite problem during their Peninsula Campaign.

NONCLASSIFIED DISEASES

The "Army Itch" plagued Yankee and Rebel alike. Over in the western theater, it was variously known as "prairie dig," "western itch," and "Missouri mange." Many believed it to be brought on by one's unhealthy constitution in contact with an irritant such as coarse-fibered clothing. But there could be no doubt that the scabies (Sarcoptes scabiei) parasite was behind it. This itch mite left its telltale fine zigzag dark burrows under the skin. The impregnated female mite laid her eggs along the tunnel. Scabies was rarely seen where regimental officers took camp hygiene seriously, and those who ignored it would find an itch of epidemic proportions racing through the ranks. After a determined bout of scratching, an added grief would present itself as a bacterial infection such as impetigo.

SARCOPTES SCABIEI

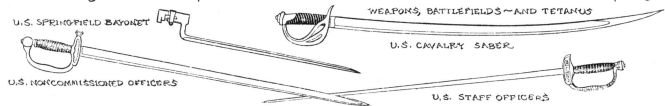

U.S. SPRINGFIELD BAYONET

U.S. NONCOMMISSIONED OFFICERS

WEAPONS, BATTLEFIELDS ~ AND TETANUS

U.S. CAVALRY SABER

U.S. STAFF OFFICERS

Tetanus, known to the troops as lockjaw, was known to originate from a wound. What wasn't known was that the battlefield was the worst place to receive one ~ and little wonder. Any open landscape suitable for military maneuvers would also be prime grazing ground for horses and cattle. There the animals would leave their droppings, rich in the spores of the Clostridium tetani. Once a soldier was gashed, punctured, or shot, that break in the skin was an open door for the bacteria to enter and multiply.

Venereal disease was no stranger to either army. Progressive purulent urethral discharge made it clear that the owner of the bacterial gonorrhea had engaged in an indiscretion. Worse yet the shady lady may have given the soldier a syphilitic chancre and a collection of swollen inguinal lymph glands. The spirochetes causing such mischief sooner or later would produce a skin rash and one day involve the brain, spinal cord, and the heart with its great vessels. Both gonorrhea and syphilis, were found to be more frequent at the beginning and at the end of the war and, understandably, more common among those stationed near cities than those on active service.

Once again prevention was the only answer in a day when treatment was a mixture of theory and medicines to counter symptoms. Certainly the poisonous mercury or iodide of potassium left much to be desired. And so in June of 1863, the Union military police at Nashville and elsewhere in Tennessee rounded up all women of "vile character" and shipped them out by riverboat to Louisville, Kentucky. Since Louisville had negative feelings on the subject, the cargo was sent along to Cincinnati. The handful of ladies who were permitted ashore were somehow ~ almost overnight ~ back in Nashville and back in business as usual. Washington ordered the remainder on shipboard to be returned to their Nashville starting point, homeward-bound, with a green light that would again turn red.

The problem was back in Nashville's lap. Desperate measures called for the hospitalization of any prostitute showing signs of a venereal disease. It seemed a workable solution to Memphis, but its provisional mayor had no wish to be associated with such goings on.

Down in Confederate country, women were not at all uncommon in the camps during the first year of the war. There were three social classes, each standing aloof from the others. The wives and daughters brought a touch of hometown respectability to camp life. Many other women worked as camp cooks and laundresses, while the third and smallest group, the "fallen women," offered a different sort of service. Hardship, improved discipline, and the order that "company laundresses who do not actually wash for men must be discharged" effectively eliminated any camp followers.

As in the Union Army, the concentration of soldiers in southern cities was a magnet for prostitutes. In the autumn of 1864, Mayor Mayo complained that "never was a place more changed than Richmond. Go on the Capital Square any afternoon, and you may see these women parading up and down the shady walks jostling respectable ladies into the gutter." One madam even opened a bawdy house across the street from a soldiers' hospital that was run by the Young Men's Christian Association. Be that as it may, it must be mentioned that the vast majority of Yankees and Rebels, like the provisional mayor of Memphis, would have nothing to do with such outlandish behavior.

Nostalgia was considered a camp disease brought on by the hardships, discomforts, and exposures of wartime. Two types of soldiers were most susceptible, according to the contemporary Medical and Surgical History of the Rebellion. One was "young men of feeble will, highly developed imaginative facilities and strong sexual desires"~ perhaps the group that gave Nashville and Memphis so many problems. And there were the "married men for the first time absent from their families."

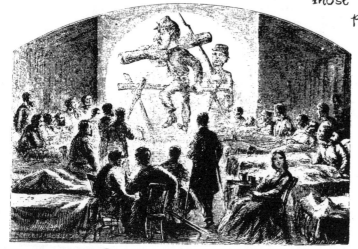

MAGIC LANTERNS IN THE HOSPITALS LESSENED NOSTALGIA

The monotony of winter camps fueled nostalgia, while active campaigning relieved "morbid depression" and restlessness in the ranks. Here again prevention was worth any pound of cure. Any thinking officer could revive the energies that languished in the winter camps. Spirits could be rejuvenated while improving camp life. Better comforts and conveniences, improved health in the fresh air through sport contests and group activities, and a more interesting variety of drills and fighting skills could be real morale boosters. As the United States Sanitary Commission stated many times, a clean, healthy, and well-adjusted soldier living in a well-policed camp might escape many of those hard-to-cure diseases (see Sidelight 16).

UTENSILS,

Apparatus, &c., for Physicians,

FOR SALE BY

BULLOCK & CRENSHAW,

Sixth Street, two doors above Arch Street,

PHILADELPHIA.

———1857———

ADHESIVE PLASTER, . . . per yard,
" " in cans of 2 yards ½ width, per can,

Fig. 1. Fig. 2.

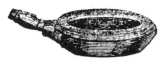

BED PANS, round and slant, Queensware, (Fig. 1 & 2,)

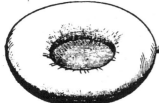

Fig. 3.

BED PANS, India rubber, inflating, (Fig. 3,)

Fig. 4.

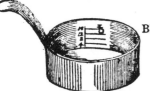

BLEEDING BOWLS, White Ware, graduated, (Fig. 4,)

CAUSTIC HOLDERS, Glass, in Morocco Case, (Fig. 10,)

Fig. 10.

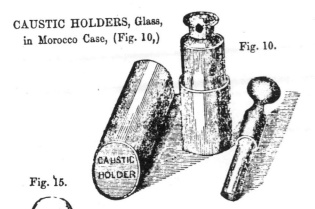

CAUSTIC HOLDER

Fig. 15.

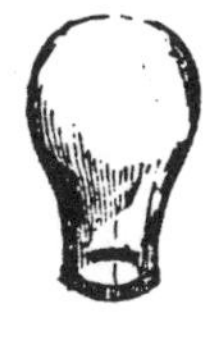

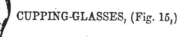

CUPPING-GLASSES, (Fig. 15,)

Fig. 32. Fig. 33.

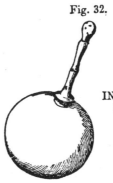

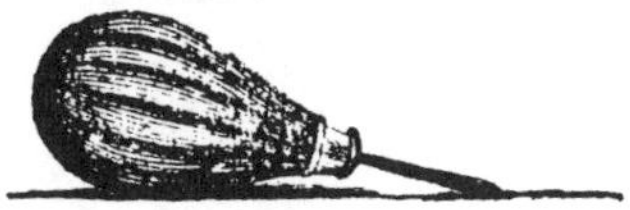

INJECTING SYRINGE, Elastic, (Fig. 32,)
Female, with Ivory Pipe,
Male, with Metal Pipe, (Fig. 33,)

Fig. 34.

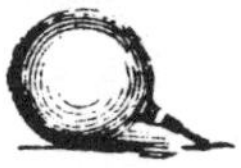

ELASTIC SYRINGE, for Ear, (Ivory Pipe,) (Fig. 34,) . . . .

Fig. 35.

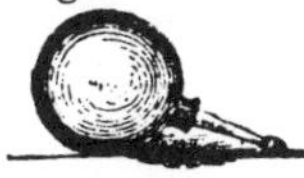

ELASTIC SYRINGE, for Penis, (Ivory Pipe, (Fig. 35,) . . .

Fig. 36. Fig. 37.

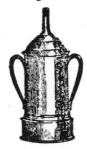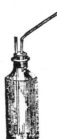

INHALERS, (Queensware,) for administering Medicated Vapors, (Fig. 36,) .

INHALERS (Glass,) (Fig. 37,) .

Fig. 89.

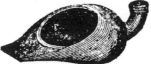

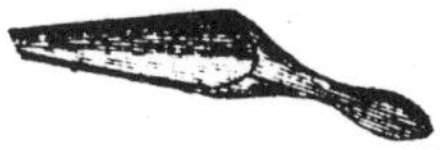

SPECULUMS, Ear, Wilde's, (Fig. 89,) . . .

SPECULUMS, German Silver, for Ear, Bivalve, .
Ear, Conical, 3 in a set, (Silver,)
" " 3 in a set, (German Silver,)

Fig. 90.

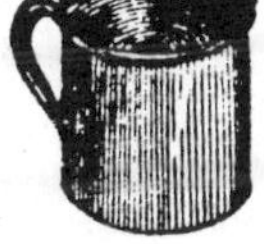

Fig. 91.

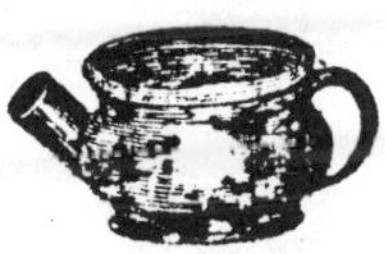

SPITTING CUPS, of Queensware, with movable tops, (Fig. 90,) .

SPITTING CUPS, with Spout, Queensware, Top movable, (Fig. 91,) . . .
STETHOSCOPES, Cedar, plain, . . .
" " Ivory mounted, .
" Ebony, plain, . .
" " Ivory mounted, .
" Ivory mounted, with Pleximeter,
STOMACH TUBES, best quality, . .
SUSPENSORY BANDAGES, Cotton, .
" " " Movable Pouch,
" " Silk, . .

Fig. 92.

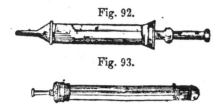

Fig. 93.

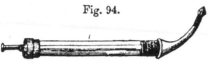

SYRINGES, Glass, Male and Female, (Figs. 92 and 93,)
"   Metal-capped, small,

Fig. 94.

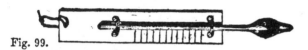

SYRINGES, Glass, Curved, for Uterus, (Fig. 94,)
"   "   "   for Ear,

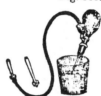

Fig. 99.

THERMOMETERS, Small, on Ivory Scale, with
Bulb projecting below the Scale, graduated
from 50° to 140° F. (Fig. 99,)

Fig. 101.

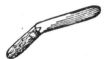

TONGUE DEPRESSERS, Pearl,
"   Steel, heavily plated with
Silver,
"   Steel, (Fig. 101,)

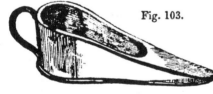

Fig. 103.

URINALS, Fe-
male, Slipper
Pattern, (Fig.
103,)

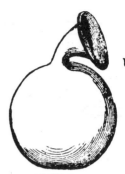

URINALS,
Glass, male
and female,
(Fig. 104,)

Fig. 104.

Fig. 111.

SYRINGE, Arnott's Elastic Self, in Morocco Case, (Fig. 111,)

Fig. 112.

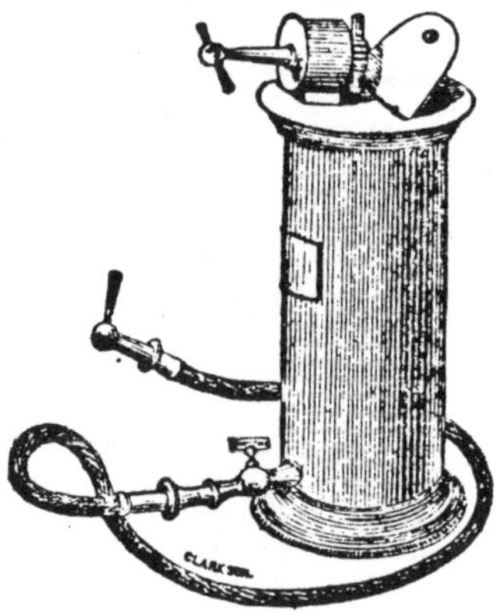

SYRINGES, French, Self-
Acting. The liquid is
introduced at once into
the Syringe, dispensing
with any other vessel.
The force is derived
from a strong spring in
the box at the top, act-
ing directly on the
plunger. The quantity,
and direction of the cur-
rent is regulated by the
stop-cock and flexible
tube at the bottom.
This Syringe is not lia-
ble to get out of order,
(Fig. 112.)

BULLOCK & CRENSHAW, PHILADELPHIA.

MAGNETO-ELECTRIC MACHINES

FOR THE APPLICATION OF ELECTRICITY FOR MEDICAL PURPOSES.

Fig. 114.

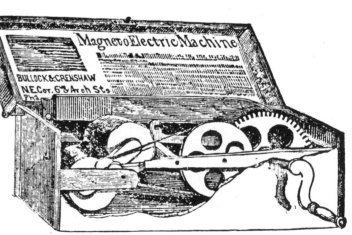

The current is derived from an armature covered with helices of fine
insulated copper wire, revolving rapidly in proximity to the poles of
a strong magnet.

This Battery has been successfully used in a number of cases of
Suspended Animation arising from narcotic poisons. In Paralysis,
Neuralgia, Rheumatism and Nervous Disorders, it has been emi-
nently serviceable.

As no Acids are required, the Battery is at any moment ready for
service. It is put in motion simply by turning the crank shown in
the figure.

A neat mahogany box, (with lock and key) 9½ inches long, by 4½
inches in width and height, contains the apparatus.

MEDICAL POISONS

The United States Sanitary Commission was right on target with its ounce of prevention being worth a pound of cure. Treatment of a disease was not without its risks, for many of the common Civil War period medicines were poisonous if taken in excess. The symptomatic treatments would follow the spectrum of hoped-for results listed here without killing the patient by overdosing in the process.

DIAPHORETICS removed poisons by perspiration.
DIURETICS increased the flow of urine.
EMETICS induced vomiting.
EXPECTORANTS produced saliva.
NARCOTICS dulled pain and induced sleep.
RUBEFACIENTS produced redness of skin with topical applications.
SEDATIVES calmed or tranquilized.
SUDORIFICS induced perspiration.

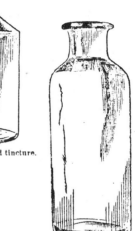

Common wide-mouth packer.

In the preparation of the potential poisons listed below, the pharmaceutical preparatory terms include
INFUSIONS ~ soaking in water to extract medicinal properties;
SOLUTIONS ~ dissolving in a liquid; and
TINCTURES ~ medicines dissolved in alcohol.

There were two kinds of such poisons: irritant poisons and narcotic poisons.

IRRITANT POISONS

These acted immediately on the digestive tract to cause vomiting, pain, and shock. ANTIMONY was used as oxide of antimony in the popular Tartar Emetic compound along with tartaric acid and potash. The white metallic-tasting crystals were used for counterirritants, emetics, rubefacients, sedatives, sudorifics, and especially for croup, colds, fevers, pneumonia, chorea ~ as well as two problems that were strangers in the military camps: difficult labors and inflamed breasts.

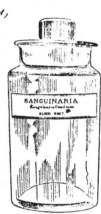

Broad German saltmouth, adapted to materia medica specimens.

ARSENIC or RAT'S-BANE was a tasteless oxidized metallic powder that was in use after workmen in a copper smelting plant were found to be free of intermittent fevers in an endemic region. It was the arsenical fumes that killed off malaria-bearing mosquitoes and not ingested arsenic as was theorized. It may well be that Confederate physicians resorted to its use in malaria when the truly curative quinine supplies were blockaded. It would be given either in pill form or dissolved in the much used Fowler's solution to produce diaphoretics and sudorifics.

American moulded tincture.

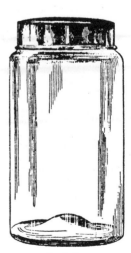

Ordinary blown tincture.   Specia Jar.

91

CANTHARIDES or SPANISH FLY, the bright green fly found in Spain, France, and Italy, was dried and powdered for topical blistering. A substitute in America and perhaps for the Southern army were the darker flies that lunched on potato and sugar beet leaves. Cantharides was also taken internally as a tincture, powder or pill for astringents, diuretics, and narcotics; it was used to treat paralysis, tetanus, diabetes, and, for the girls they left behind, it was used for suppressing menstrual periods.

NARCOTIC POISONS

Narcotic poisons took some time to be absorbed before producing symptoms, and therefore it became too late for emptying the stomach. Unconsciousness, coma, and death would not be far behind.

ACONITE or WOLFSBANE ~ the Monkshood plant in the forests of Europe with its handsome purple flowers looked innocent enough, but the leaves could be deadly if not well cooked. In times past it was given to criminals sentenced to death. Its more conventional uses included anodynes, diaphoretics, and sedatives.

BELLADONNA ~ the leaves or berries of the Deadly Nightshade, if given in too large a dose, produced stupor, delirium, convulsions, and death. These were exactly the symptoms "prescribed" for the Danish army that invaded Scotland. At a truce meeting, the Scottish hosts gave the enemy the juice of the belladonna berries mixed with wine. The invaders were very nearly exterminated. More kindly uses were counterirritants, diaphoretics, narcotics, and rubefacients in extract containing the active principle of atropine.

CAMPHOR ~ this volatile oil from the Laurus camphora, or spicewood, trees from the Far East was given in the form of a tincture or powder as a stimulant, anodyne, and expectorant, and in just about any other form when the diagnosis or treatment was in doubt.

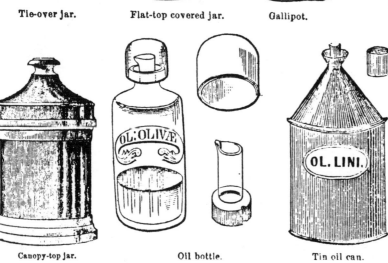

Tie-over jar. **Flat-top covered jar.** **Gallipot.**

DIGITALIS ~ the white-to-purple bell-shaped flowers of the foxglove plants (the name reflects the finger-in-a-glove appearance) that beautify many a garden. A rapid drying of the leaves preserved the medicinal potency.

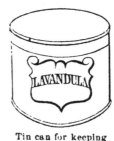

OL: OLIVÆ

OL. LINI.

LAVANDULA

Canopy-top jar. **Oil bottle.** **Tin oil can.** **Tin can for keeping herbs.**

It was used as a diuretic, narcotic, and a sedative and for reducing the force and frequency of the pulse. With excessive dosage, however, the pulse became slow and irregular accompanied by vomiting, vertigo, and death. Tinctures, infusions and powders of digitalis were available. It is still a drug much used today to make the body's pumping system more efficient.

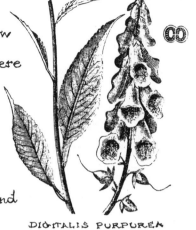

DIGITALIS PURPUREA

ERGOT ~ Fungus on the heads of rye grass, as well as barley and wheat, provided the means for stopping some hemorrhages by causing muscle spasm as an astringent.

HEMLOCK ~ The leaves and seeds of this plant found in European Mediterranean countries were gathered before flowering. Their juice provided a narcotic effect as a substitute for opium, and in the treatment of ulcers, sores, and erysipelas.

MANDRAKE or MAY APPLE ~ its oval, lemon-colored fruit ripened in late summer (not in May!) The root was used first by the American Indians as a cathartic, for intestinal worms, and, when the fresh root juice was applied to the ear, deafness. Its main use in the Civil War was as a laxative.

MERCURY or QUICKSILVER ~ its toxic properties were discovered when mercury bottles leaked in the hold of a ship and killed off the stowaway rats. Chloride of mercury, otherwise known as calomel, was something of an anti-inflammatory cure-all. It found use in rheumatic and heart diseases, restoring organs to their original condition, and in inflammatory diseases such as yellow fever, typhoid, and cholera. The symptoms of diarrhea and gastric irritability were indications for calomel. Apparently itching, chafing, and fungal scalp infections also yielded to this poisonous medicine. The first hint of overdosage might be "mercurial trembling," which was common among those who silvered mirrors.

OPIUM ~ The juice from the seed capsules of the Asian white poppy produced a tincture that American doctors called "laudanum." It was considered the best of all anodynes and sedatives available, and it was given for cholera as well.

STRYCHNINE ~ The seeds from the Strychnos nux vomica tree of India produced a tincture that was safer to use than pills. The slightly bitter elongated crystals were sold in large quantities during the Civil War period to kill crows and small critters. Small doses were used as diaphoretics and as diuretics, tonics, and laxatives. Overdoses caused the motor nerves to produce tetanuslike symptoms with generalized muscle spasm, which finally resulted in the cessation of respiration.

The general therapy for poisoning from drug overdose would be prompt use of a stomach pump, pulverized animal charcoal, milk and water, magnesia, or either mucilaginous or oily substances to protect and sooth the intestinal lining.

SOME PHARMACEUTICAL CATALOGUE OFFERINGS AT THE OUTSET OF THE CIVIL WAR

CATALOGUE

BULLOCK & CRENSHAW, PHILADELPHIA.

1857

Fig. 5.

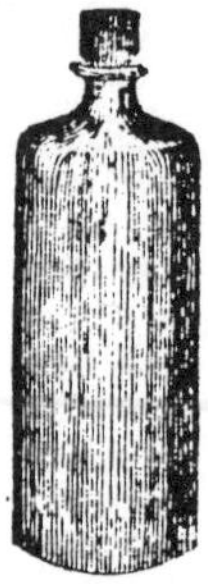

BOTTLES, Flint Glass, Narrow Mouth, with Stoppers accurately ground, (Fig. 5,)

1 gallon,
half gallon,
quart,
pint,
half pint,
4 oz.,
2 oz.,
1 oz.,
half oz.,

Fig. 6.

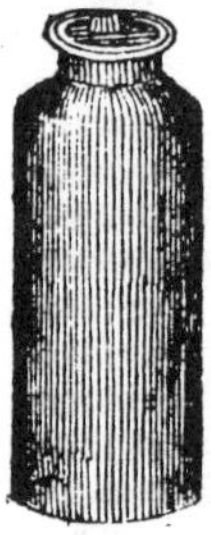

BOTTLES, Flint Glass, Wide Mouth, with Glass Stoppers, (Fig. 6,)

gallon,
half gallon,
quart,
pint,
half pint,
4 oz.,
2 oz.,
1 oz.,
half oz.,

CORKS, Vial, (Velvet) assorted,
" Pint,
" Quart,

Fig. 11.

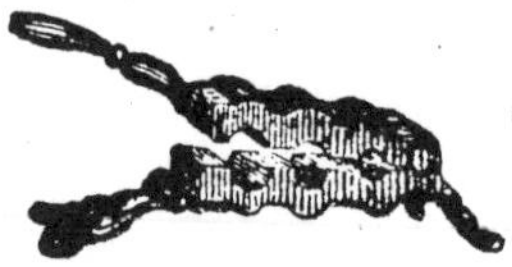

CORK PRESSES, (Fig. 11,)

CORK DRAWERS, for removing corks from inside of bottles,

Fig. 12.

Fig. 13.

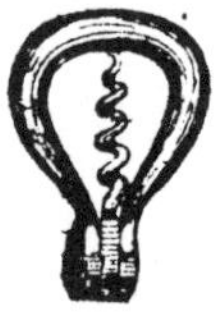

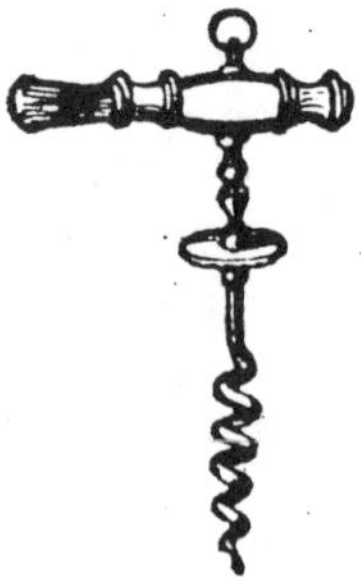

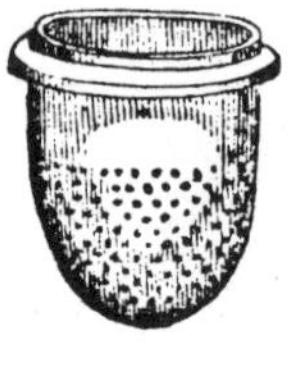

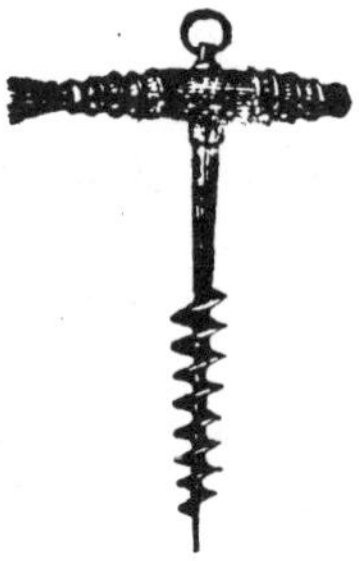

Fig. 14.

CORK-SCREW, White Bone Handle, (Fig. 12,)
" " Wood Handle, (Fig. 13,)
" " Pocket, (Fig. 14,)

Fig. 31.

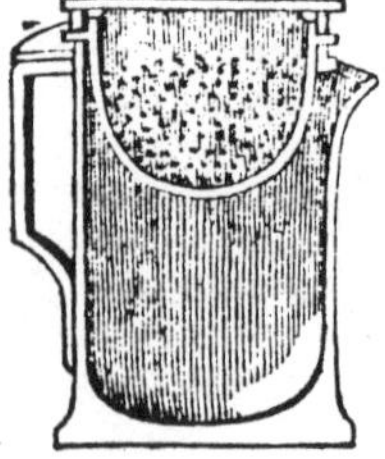

31.

INFUSION MUGS, (of White Ware,) for making Infusions, and preparing Tinctures, by circulatory displacement, (Fig. 31,)

pint,
quart,
half gallon,

MARSHE'S ARSENIC APPARATUS, (Fig. 47,)

Fig. 47.

Fig. 48.

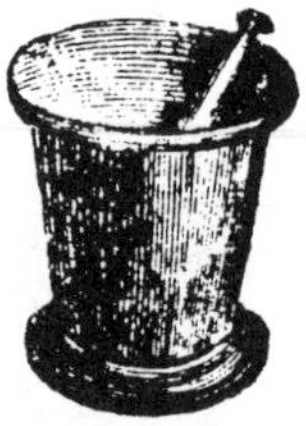

MORTARS, IRON, turned smooth on the inside, (Fig. 48,)

4 inches across top,
5 " " "
6 " " "
7 " " "
9 " " "

Fig. 49.

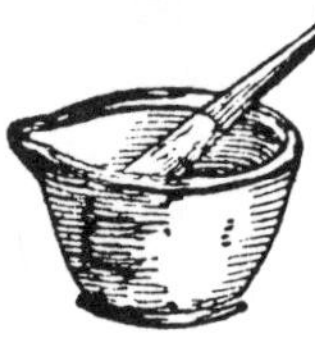

MORTARS, WEDGWOOD, (Fig. 49,)

No. 000, 2 oz.,
00, 3 oz.,
0, 4 oz.,
1, 6 oz.,
2, 8 oz.,
3, 12 oz.,
4, pint,
6, quart,
8, half-gall.,

Fig. 64.

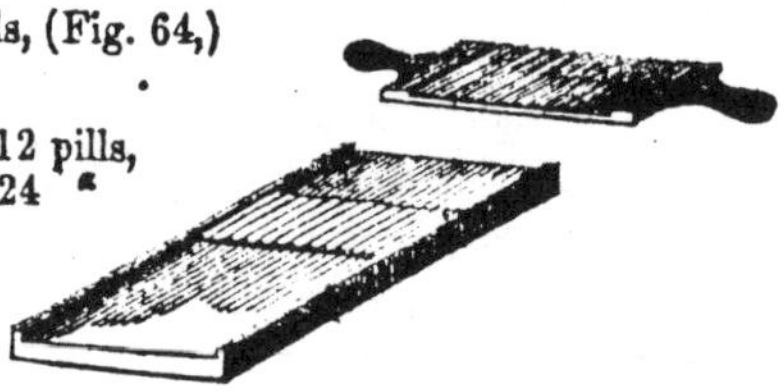

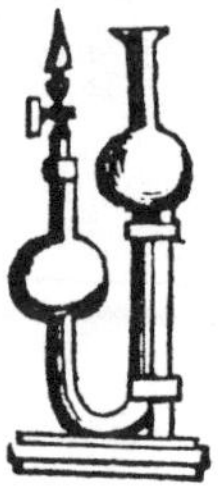

PILL MACHINES, Brass, for 12 pills, (Fig. 64,)
" " 24 "

PILL MACHINES, Wooden, for 12 pills,
" " 24 "

Fig. 65.

Fig. 66.

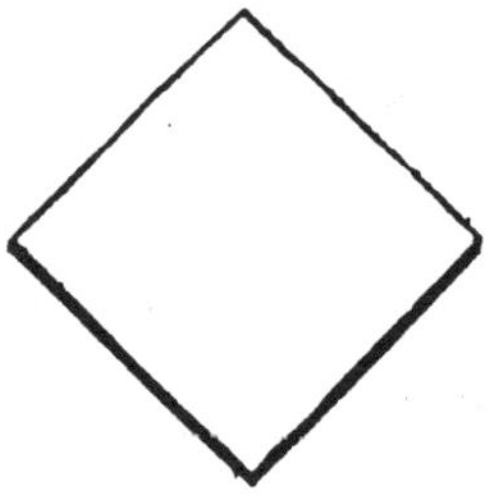

TILES, for Pills, Graduated, (Fig. 65,)

12 inches square,
8 " "
5 " "

" Plain, for Ointments, (Fig. 66,)

8 inches square,

Fig. 67.

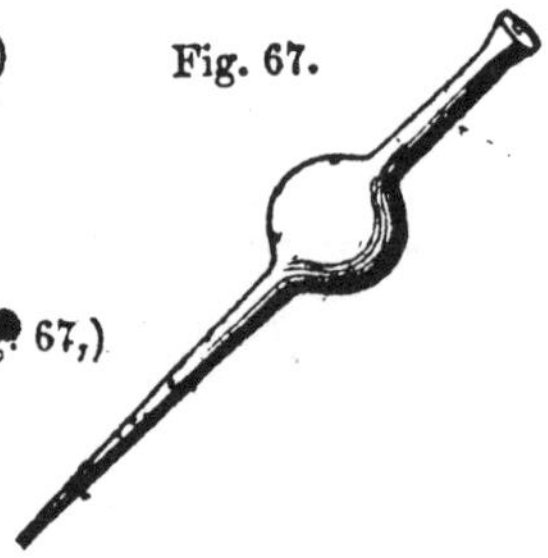

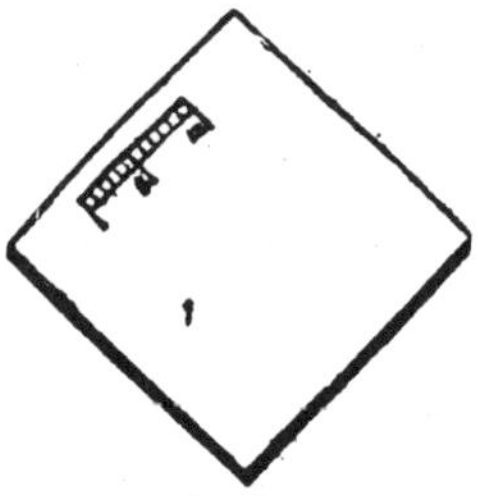

PIPETTES, or Dropping Tubes, (Fig. 67,)

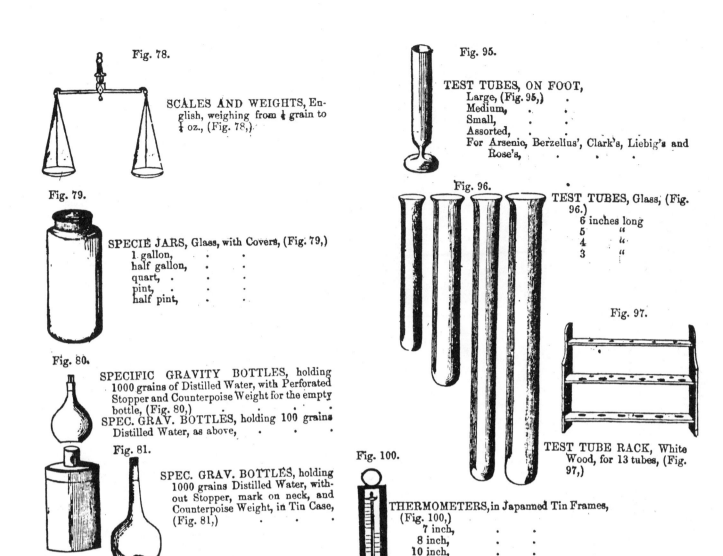

Fig. 78.

SCALES AND WEIGHTS, English, weighing from ¼ grain to ¼ oz., (Fig. 78,)

Fig. 79.

SPECIE JARS, Glass, with Covers, (Fig. 79,)
    1 gallon,
    half gallon,
    quart,
    pint,
    half pint,

Fig. 80.

SPECIFIC GRAVITY BOTTLES, holding 1000 grains of Distilled Water, with Perforated Stopper and Counterpoise Weight for the empty bottle, (Fig. 80,)
SPEC. GRAV. BOTTLES, holding 100 grains Distilled Water, as above,

Fig. 81.

SPEC. GRAV. BOTTLES, holding 1000 grains Distilled Water, without Stopper, mark on neck, and Counterpoise Weight, in Tin Case, (Fig. 81,)

Fig. 95.

TEST TUBES, ON FOOT,
    Large, (Fig. 95,)
    Medium,
    Small,
    Assorted,
    For Arsenic, Berzelius', Clark's, Liebig's and Rose's,

Fig. 96.

TEST TUBES, Glass, (Fig. 96.)
    6 inches long
    5 "
    4 "
    3 "

Fig. 97.

TEST TUBE RACK, White Wood, for 13 tubes, (Fig. 97,)

Fig. 100.

THERMOMETERS, in Japanned Tin Frames, (Fig. 100,)
    7 inch,
    8 inch,
    10 inch,
    12 inch,

HAMMOND VS. MERCURIAL POISONS

In May of 1863 Surgeon General Hammond received a disturbing report concerning Grant's troops' march on Vicksburg. One of his medical inspectors had found an excessive number of salivation cases from those old standby favorites, calomel and tartar emetic. These mercury-laced poisons had the potential effect of soldiers losing their teeth or even mercurial gangrine if they were overdosed.

Hammond promptly removed these dangers from the army's supply table and was roundly applauded by such notables as Dr. Oliver Wendell Holmes. Unfortunately, their approval was countered by an uprising among the run-of-the-mill physicians. Their voices were joined by a battery of old enemies of Hammond and the Sanitary Commission, including Secretary of War Stanton. By the summer of 1863 they had moved in for the kill, and Hammond had lost his surgeon generalship to Dr. Joseph Barnes.

Hammond's lasting credits included working with Letterman to reorganize the ambulance service and the field and general hospitals; to provide trained nursing care; and to establish an overall quality upgrading

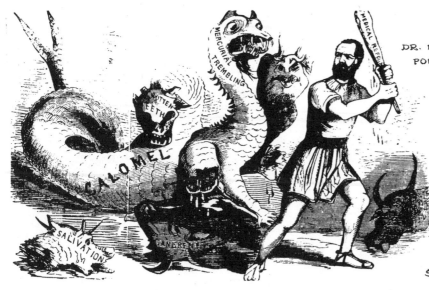

of all physicians and surgeons entering the service. One of his first innovations in 1862 was to ready enough medical supplies to last 100,000 soldiers for half a year. Stockpiling these supplies for future camp epidemics or extended campaigns had never seemed to enter the heads of the previous surgeon generals.

MEDICAL SUPPLIES

As the war progressed, the cost of medicines rose with the demand. Sometimes the supplies were of questionable quality. In the fall of 1862, Hammond let it be known that he was considering establishing federal drug laboratories in Philadelphia and New York to provide the army with quality medicines at minimal cost.

It may have been nothing more than a bluff~ but it worked. The large pharmaceutical laboratories such as Wyeth, Squibb, and Pfizer soon dropped prices to rock bottom rather than lose their lucrative army sales. The savings to the war effort were considerable.

The Confederacy considered the need for medicines and medical supplies second only to weapons and clothing. With most of the pharmaceutical companies in the North, stockpiling began before war was declared. As the blockade of Southern ports became more effective, any civilian use of medicines needed by the Rebel army was prohibited. The capture of any Yankee supplies was welcomed but of little lasting benefit.

Southern resourcefulness was the answer. Along every roadside and in field and woodland grew plants long used as medicinals by the country folk and the Indians who preceded them. Surgeon General Moore delegated Dr. Francis P. Porcher of Charleston to investigate these potential medicines. The result was the

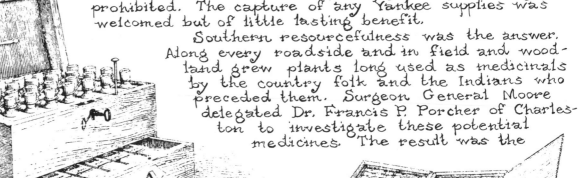

doctor's highly regarded book <u>Resources of Southern Fields and Forests</u>, printed in 1863. Newly organized laboratories began turning out of substitute treatments, many with a greater degree of safety than the usual symptomatic sovereign remedies.

Many a Rebel letter from camp made mention of such foraged medicinals. Diarrhea and malaria were dosed with a hot tea made from the bark of slippery elm, sweet gum, willow, and dogwood, while measles patients took a drink brewed of spice wood. Fleas apparently beat a hasty retreat from fresh pennyroyal leaves being sewed in a bag and placed in the soldier's bed. There were many vegetable substitute cathartics, but to control overactive intestines there was also blackberry, willow, and sweet gum bark for the taking. The troops brought in their own scurvy cures in the form of wild onion, garlic, mustard, sassafras, pokeweed, artichoke, pepper grass and dandelion greens. Vinegar was also used. Itch sufferers received a poke-root solution internally and as an ointment. One physician reported excellent results with urethral injections of ink ball. Further, a substitute for quinine was a tonic of native barks and whiskey.

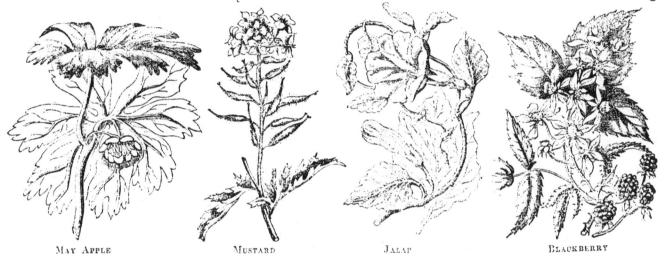

MAY APPLE   MUSTARD   JALAP   BLACKBERRY

Blockades were nondiscriminatory, for much-needed quinine, morphine, smallpox vaccines, chloroform, and ether were blocked along with the weapons for making war. Certainly, no right-thinking American would purposely deprive the sick and wounded of any pharmaceuticals or surgical supplies. In the 1945 "House of Squibb" monograph, it was recorded that Squibb not only supplied many medicines to the Union Army but "indirectly he met the needs of the Confederates as well, for a good share of his ether found its way into Southern lines. It was even said that Abraham Lincoln himself chose to overlook the smuggling of Squibb ether to the South." Certainly many a drug or can of ether was smuggled across the lines under hats and petticoats.

THE AFTERMATH Wrong!

On April 9, 1865, four years of bloody conflict ended when Lee surrendered the Confederate Army to Grant at the Appomattox Court House. President Lincoln now faced the awesome task of rebuilding his shattered country into a truly united states of America. In his second inaugural address, he emphasized a "just and lasting peace with malice toward none and charity for all." Five days later at 10:30 in the evening, as he watched a play at Ford's Theater, a demented actor fired his der-

DERRINGER

ringer point-blank at the back of the president's head. The one leader who could smooth the road to a reconstruction of a battered South now lay close to death.

"The Medical and Surgical Reporter" of Philadelphia in its April 22, 1865 edition gave the details of all that followed (see Sidelight 17 for Lincoln's autopsy). Under the direction of Assistant Surgeons Charles A. Leale, U.S.V. and C.S. Taft, U.S.A., the unconscious president was rushed to the nearest private house. There an examination with the finger introduced into the oozing occipital wound (for this natural probe was considered proper in that presterilization era) found the bullet beyond reach. Lincoln's breathing was labored, and there were the ominous signs of the left pupil contraction and right pupil dilatation. Neither reacted to light.

Surgeon General Barnes and Lincoln's family physician Dr. Robert K. Stone, arrived to take charge. The only surgical procedure during that long night was the periodic removal of clot formations from the wound that were causing an irregular pulse. About 2:00 A.M. the surgeon general searched the wound with a silver probe and found a plug of occipital bone lodged in the projectile's path. With a longer Nélaton probe (see page 46) he was able to bypass the obstruction and locate the bullet in the right anterior lobe of the cerebrum. The white porcelain tip of the probe failed to pick up the telltale lead marks transferred from the bullet because of its unusual hardness.

The death watch continued "with all the leading men of the profession in the city in attendance" until death came at 7:22 A.M. on April 15th. An autopsy five hours later found that the flattened spherical bullet had coursed from left to the right front of the brain, splintering both orbital plates. With such great damage, "it was the opinion of the surgeons in charge that most patients would have died in two hours from the reception of such an injury."

THE MAKE-DO SURGICAL SET- Surgeon General Barnes, along with some of his Medical Bureau staff~ Colonel Crane, and Doctors Stone, Woodward, Curtis, Notson, and Taft were responsible for their president's autopsy. The uncertainty and concern that permeated all Washington were translated into a sense of urgency for the autopsy team. They gathered without one very necessary item: an autopsy set. No matter ~ one of their number offered his private surgical set as a substitute. Meanwhile a young army surgeon of lowly rank, Dr. Alfred D. Wilson, was on detached duty and working under the surgeon general. He was given the chore of guarding the door to the autopsy room. When the chosen few had finished, one of the surgeons ~ we know not which one ~ gave his just-used surgical set to Wilson. Perhaps it was a consolation prize for his missing so extraordinary an event.

But Wilson was also well aware that he was in possession of a most important piece of medical history. With time the mahogany case with its instruments by various makers came down through the family. It was presented to the Medical Society of the County of Kings, Brooklyn, New York at their May 20, 1935 meeting.

AND IN CONCLUSION

Dr. Timothy Childs, who began these pages with his remarks to the 1856-57 medical school class, was right on target. He had concluded that "medicine does improve, but it improves slowly." A prompt rethinking of the popular medical theories was long overdue. The germ theory had been laughed off as an outlandish notion, and "inflammations," childhood diseases, and camp fevers would continue to be treated symptomatically. It remained the gospel that any injury or stimulation of the senses or emotions, or breathing tainted air could throw the body's functions out of equilibrium. Cathartics, diaphoretics, counterirritants, sedation, and an appropriate diet would readjust the imbalance and their symptoms.

You may remember Dr. Ignaz Semmelweiss, the Hungarian obstetrician who received more than his share of grief when he insisted that all hands, instruments, and wards should be scrubbed clean before every delivery. Had the medical world listened, many thousands of America's Civil War soldiers would not have died from septic surgery. It was somewhat ironic that the same year that the conflict ended, Scotland's Dr. Joseph Lister proved again that using an antiseptic carbolic acid spray in the operating room could save lives and prevent the usual pus-ridden complications. The germ theory was beginning to make sense.

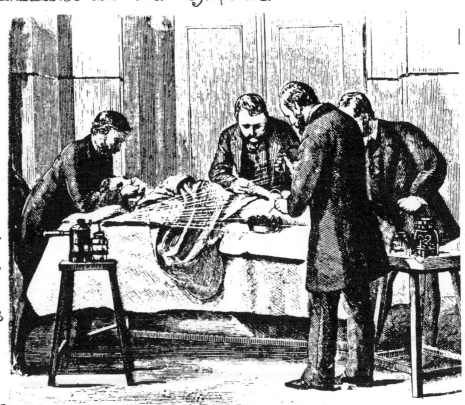

DR. JOSEPH LISTER'S CARBOLIC SPRAY STERILIZER

Thereafter medical improvements came more rapidly - and with some breathtaking discoveries. The year after Lister's surgical triumph, Louis Pasteur discovered that microscopic organisms were responsible for turning fermenting wine into vinegar. His solution was simple enough: destroy the offenders by heating, otherwise known as pasteurization. He went on in 1881 to show that modified heat could attenuate the virulence of anthrax. When these tamed bacteria were injected into a patient, the body responded by building up an immunity to the disease. This success was followed two years later by giving preventive injections against rabies. Robert Koch followed up by identifying

99

tubular-shaped bacteria as the cause of tuberculosis. The new science of bacteriology was off and running, and the germ theory had been proven beyond a shadow of a doubt.

Unfortunately these discoveries came too late to call a halt to the innumerable amputations that prevented a spreading infection. These and any deaths from disease could be only somewhat influenced by preventative measures. Through the trial-and-error experiences in the Revolutionary War and the later Crimean War, personal hygiene, enforced camp sanitation, and the pavilion hospital concept helped to reduce the number of war deaths. The United States Sanitary Commission watchdogs deserved the gratitude of the Northern families back home for keeping their sons in uniform healthy. Even so, germ-causing disease claimed slightly more than two Union deaths for every life lost on the battlefield. Although the Confederate records were lost in the Richmond fires, it has been estimated that the toll approached a ratio of three infection deaths to one lost to weapons.

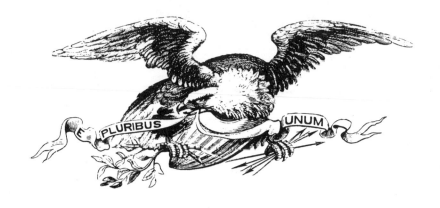

The old military saying that an army must know and understand its enemy for a successful campaign holds true for medicine. By the Spanish American War, doctors were more aware of and better prepared to combat their microscopic foes.

Meanwhile the regular and volunteer physicians and the surgeons of the Civil War were themselves targets of both bacteria and bullets. On the Union side 32 were killed in battle, or by guerillas or partizans, and 9 by accidents; 83 were wounded in action, of whom 10 died; 4 died in Rebel prisons, 7 of yellow fever, 3 of cholera, and 271 of other diseases, most of which were incidental to camp life or the result of exposure in the field. The Confederate physician and surgeon losses are unknown. All had made the ultimate sacrifice while pursuing their profession and their convictions.

Sidelights

Sidelight 1

General McClellan heartily endorsed the effort of the Ladies' Aid Society of Philadelphia to make slippers for the sick and wounded Union soldiers. Such footwear would ward off illness with warm feet—and at no cost. A sewing pattern was provided for Northern housewives to cut and stitch each pair from leftover fabric. The women were confident that "according to actual trial a pair of slippers can be completed in neat workmanlike manner in one hour."

Source: Civilization: The Magazine of the Library of Congress, *vol. 3, no. 4 (Aug.-Sept. 1996)*

Sidelight 2

The origin of Taps

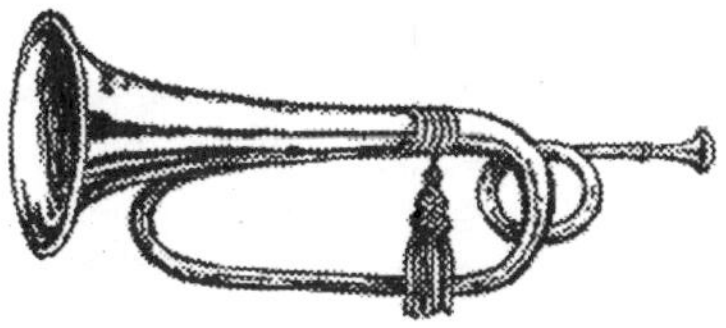

The Union Army's Peninsula Campaign had met stubborn resistance during the Battle of Seven Days. Colonel Daniel Butterfield had been wounded in an early engagement at Gaines' Mills, and, while recuperating, he jotted down on an old envelope a new bugle call. He hoped it would be a more quieting evening call when the heavy fighting was over.

That night came the first week of July 1862 as the Army of the Potomac rested at Harrison's Landing by the James River. The colonel whistled the tune to the bugler, and shortly the entire camp heard and liked the first sounding of Taps. They were not alone. The call was adopted by the entire Union army. The Confederates did so after hearing taps—from a distance, of course—instead of a volley at one of the Union funerals. The Rebels honored Stonewall Jackson the same way when he was laid to rest in 1863.

Sidelight 3

UNION AND CONFEDERATE ARMY UNITS
COMPANY = 100 soldiers commanded by 2 captains
REGIMENT = 10 companies of 300–1,000 soldiers commanded by a colonel
BRIGADE = 2–5 regiments of 1,000–4,000 soldiers commanded by a brigadier general
DIVISION = 2–5 brigades of 4,000–12,000 soldiers commanded by a major general
CORPS = 3–4 divisions of 23,000–40,000 soldiers commanded by a Union major general or a Confederate lieutenant general

Sidelight 4

The surgical instruments carried in the Autenreith Medicine wagon were:

The *Capital Operating Case* contained: 2 amputating knives (one long, one medium), 2 catlings (one long, one medium), 4 scalpels, 1 cartilage knife, 1 capital saw (long, bow, two blades), 1 metacarpal saw, 1 chain saw, 1 Hey's saw, 1 trephine (conical), 1 trephine (small crown), 1 bone forceps (Liston's long, sharp, spring handle), 1 bone forceps (broad edge, slightly curved, spring handle), 1 bone forceps (gnawing, spring handle), 1 bone forceps (sequestrum, spring handle), 1 artery forceps, 1 artery needle, 1 artery needle key, 12 surgeon's needles, 1 tourniquet screw with pad, 1 tenaculum, 1 scissors, 1 chisel, 1 gouge, 1 mallet, 4 drills (with one handle), 2 retractors, 1 raspatory, 1 elevator, 1 brush, 12 yards suture wire (iron), ¼ oz. ligature silk, ⅛ oz. wax, 1 mahogany case (brass bound, slide catch), 1 leather pouch.

The *Minor Operating Case* contained: 1 amputating knife, 3 scalpels, 2 bistouries, 1 hernia knife, 1 finger knife, 1 artery forceps, 1 ball forceps, 1 gullet forceps, 1 dressing forceps, 1 dissection forceps, 1 artery needle, 1 artery needle key, 12 surgeon's needles, 1 tenaculum, 2 scissors, 1 trocar and canula, 1 Belloc's canula, 1 bullet probe, 1 director, 1 cutting pliers (small), 6 steel bougies (silvered, double curve, Nos. 1 and 2, 3 and 4, 5 and 6, 7 and 8, 9 and 10, 11 and 12), 3 silver catheters (Nos. 3, 6, and 9), 6 gum-elastic catheters (Nos. 1, 3, 5, 7, 9, and 11), 24 suture pins (silvered), 6 yards suture wire (iron), ¼ oz. ligature silk, ⅛ oz. wax, 1 mahogany case (brass bound, slide catch), 1 leather pouch.

The *Pocket Case* contained: 1 scalpel, 3 bistouries, 1 tentome, 1 gum lancet, 2 thumb lancets, 1 razor (small), 1 artery forceps, 1 dressing forceps, 1 artery needle, 6 surgeon's needles, 1 exploring needle, 1 tenaculum, 1 scissors, 1 director, 3 probes, 1 caustic holder, 1 silver catheter (compound), 6 yards suture wire (iron), ¼ oz. ligature silk, ⅛ oz. wax, 1 Russia leather case.

The *Field Case* contained: 2 amputating knives (one long, one medium), 2 catlings (one long, one medium), 3 scalpels, 2 bistouries, 1 hernia knife, 1 finger knife, 1 capital saw (long, bow, two blades), 1 metacarpal saw, 1 Hey's saw, 1 trephine (conical), 1 bone forceps (broad edged, slightly curved, spring handle), 1 bone forceps (sequestrum, spring handle), 1 artery forceps, 1 ball forceps, 1 dressing forceps, 1 dissection forceps, 1 artery needle, 1 artery needle key, 12 surgeon's needles, 1 tourniquet screw with pad, 1 tenaculum, 2 scissors, 2 retractors, 1 trocar and canula, 1 raspatory, 1 elevator, 1 brush, 1 bullet probe, 1 director, 6 steel bougies, (silvered, double curve, Nos. 1 and 2, 3 and 4, 5 and 6, 7 and 8, 9 and 10, 11 and 12), 3 silver catheters (Nos. 3, 6, and 9), 6 gum-elastic catheters (Nos. 1, 3, 5, 7, 9, and 11), 12 yards suture wire (iron), ¼ oz. ligature silk, ½ oz. wax, 1 mahogany case (brass bound, slide catch), 1 leather pouch; pocket case the same as allowed to staff surgeons.

CONSOLIDATED STATEMENT OF ARTICLES OF MEDICAL AND HOSPITAL PROPERTY CARRIED
WITH THE ARMY OF THE POTOMAC ACROSS THE RAPIDAN (MAY 4, 1864).*

Drugs

Acacia	Ammonium carbonate	Collodion	Whiskey
Sulfuric acid	Ammonia water	Ferric chloride	Brandy
Tannic acid	Spirits of ammonia	Mercury pills	Lead acetate
Tartaric acid	Silver nitrate	Morphine	Potassium arsenite
Ether	Camphor	Olive oil	Potassium iodide
Alcohol	Cantharides	Castor oil	Quinine
Alum	Chloroform (35 quarts)	Turpentine	Liquid soap
		Opium	Squill

*Official Records

Source:"Medicine of the Civil War" booklet published by the National Library of Medicine

Sidelight 5

CONFEDERATE MEDICINE WAGON*

Acetic acid	Arsenic oxide	Digitalis	Opium
Adhesive plaster	Assafoetida	Ether	Quinine sulphate
Alcohol	Columbo	Hydrochloric acid	Rhubarb
Aloes	Copaiba	Hyoscyamus	Senna
Ammonia water	Creosote	Morphine sulfate	Sugar
			Sulfuric acid

*Official Records

Source:"Medicine of the Civil War" booklet published by the National Library of Medicine

Sidelight 6

Summary of Nine Hundred and Twenty-two Sabre and Bayonet Wounds recorded during the American Civil War, 1861–65.

SEAT OF INJURY.	TOTAL NUMBER OF CASES.	SABRE.					BAYONET.				
		Cases.	Recoveries.	Fatal.	Undetermined Results.	Mortality.	Cases.	Recoveries.	Fatal.	Undetermined Results.	Mortality.
Sabre and Bayonet Wounds of Scalp	300	282	276	6	.....	2.1	18	16	2	.....	11.1
Sabre and Bayonet Fractures of Cranium	55	49	36	13	.....	26.5	6	1	5	.....	83.3
Sabre and Bayonet Wounds of Face	64	37	33	1	3	2.9	27	22	1	4	43.4
Sabre and Bayonet Wounds of Neck	9	5	4	.....	1	.....	4	3	1	.....	25.0
Sabre and Bayonet Wounds of Chest	38	9	8	1	.....	11.1	29	18	9	2	33.3
Sabre and Bayonet Wounds of Abdominal Parietes	18	2	2	.....	.....	.....	16	16	.....	.....	.....
Penetrations of Abdominal Cavity without injury to Viscera	10	1	.....	1	.....	100.0	9	6	3	.....	33.3
Penetrations of Abdominal Cavity with injury to Viscera	7	4	2	2	.....	50.0	3	2	1	.....	33.3
Sabre and Bayonet Wounds of the Pelvis	9	1	1	.....	.....	.....	8	6	2	.....	25.0
Sabre and Bayonet Wounds of the Back	34	13	13	.....	.....	.....	21	21	.....	.....	.....
Sabre and Bayonet Flesh Wounds of Upper Extremities	149	80	75	1	4	1.3	69	61	1	7	1.6
Sabre and Bayonet Fractures of Clavicle or Scapula	7	4	4	.....	.....	.....	3	3	.....	.....	.....
Sabre and Bayonet Wounds of Elbow Joint	9	6	6	.....	.....	.....	3	3	.....	.....	.....
Sabre Wounds of Bones of Forearm	7	7	6	1	.....	14.2	.....	.....	.....	.....	.....
Sabre and Bayonet Flesh Wounds of Lower Extremities	198	22	22	.....	.....	.....	176	171	5	.....	2.8
Bayonet Wounds of the Knee Joint	7	.....	.....	.....		.....	7	7	.....	.....	.....
Bayonet Wounds of the Metatarsals	1	.....	.....	.....		.....	1	1	.....	.....	.....
Aggregates	922	522	488	26	8	5.0	400	357	30	13	7.7

Tabular Statement of the Shot Wounds of the Upper and Lower Extremities recorded during the American Civil War.

NATURE AND SEAT OF INJURY.	Cases.	RESULTS. Recoveries.	Deaths.	Undeterm'd Results.	Percentage of Fatality.
SHOT WOUNDS OF THE UPPER EXTREMITIES.					
Flesh Wounds of the Upper Extremities ....54,729 ⎫	54,801	53,095	1,634	....	2.9
Periarticular Wounds of the Shoulder Joint..............72 ⎭		66	6	....	8.3
Fractures of the Clavicle and Scapula.............	2,280	1,936	314	30	13.9
Fractures of the Bones of the Shoulder Joint................	1,378	916	449	13	32.8
Fractures of the Bones of the Shoulder Joint in Confederate Army (excisions) ...	201	32	43	126	57.3
Fractures and Contusions of the Shaft of the Humerus................	8,245	6,249	1,639	357	20.7
Fractures of the Bones of the Elbow Joint.................	2,678	2,130	513	35	19.4
Fractures of the Bones of the Elbow Joint in the Confederate Army (excisions).	138	81	19	38	19.0
Fractures and Contusions of the Bones of the Forearm................	5,194	4,636	482	76	9.4
Fractures and Contusions of the Bones of the Wrist Joint................	1,496	1,292	193	11	12.9
Fractures of the Bones of the Wrist Joint in the Confederate Army (excisions)...	13	13	....	....	....
Fractures and Contusions of the Bones of the Hand	11,369	9,644	316	1,409	3.1
Total Shot Wounds of Upper Extremities................	87,793	80,090	5,608	2,095	6.5
SHOT WOUNDS OF THE LOWER EXTREMITIES.					
Flesh Wounds of the Lower Extremities ....58,702 ⎫	59,139	55,914	2,788	....	4.7
Periarticular Wounds of the Hip, Knee, and Ankle Joints ....437 ⎭		305	132	....	30.2
Fractures of the Bones of the Hip Joint................	386	59	327	....	84.7
Contusions of the Shaft of the Femur................	162	120	42	....	25.9
Fractures of the Shaft of the Femur................	6,576	2,995	3,392	189	53.1
Contusions of the Bones of the Knee Joint................	43	24	19	....	44.1
Fractures of the Bones of the Knee Joint................	3,355	1,542	1,800	13	53.8
Contusions of the Bones of the Leg................	183	157	26	....	14.2
Fractures of the Bones of the Leg................	8,988	6,334	2,376	278	27.2
Contusions of the Bones of the Ankle Joint................	11	8	3	....	27.2
Fractures of the Bones of the Ankle Joint................	1,711	1,239	457	15	26.9
Contusions of the Bones of the Foot................	27	26	1	....	3.7
Fractures of the Bones of the Foot................	5,832	4,942	450	440	8.3
Total Shot Wounds of Lower Extremities................	86,413	73,665	11,813	935	13.8

Sidelight 7

Tabular Statement of Twenty-nine Thousand Nine Hundred and Eighty Amputations, indicating Seat of Operation and Results.

AMPUTATIONS	CASES. Totals.	Recoveries.	Deaths.	Results Unknown.	Percentage of Fatality.
UPPER EXTREMITIES					
Amputations of the Hand or Fingers................	7,902	6,551	198	1,153	2.9
Amputations of the Wrist Joint................	68	60	7	1	10.4
Amputations in the Forearm	1,761	1,503	245	13	14.0
Amputation at the Elbow Joint................	40	36	3	1	7.6
Amputations in the Upper Arm................	5,510	4,054	1,273	183	23.8
Amputations at the Shoulder Joint................	866	596	245	25	29.1
LOWER EXTREMITIES					
Amputations of the Foot or Toes................	1,519	1,317	81	121	5.7
Amputations at the Ankle Joint................	161	119	40	2	25.1
Amputations in the Leg	5,523	3,595	1,790	138	33.2
Amputations at the Knee Joint................	195	82	111	2	57.5
Amputations in the Thigh................	6,369	2,878	3,411	80	54.2
Amputations at the Hip Joint................	66	11	55	....	83.3
Aggregates................	29,980	20,082	7,459	1,719	26.3

Sidelight 8

Table indicating Percentage of Fatality and Relative Frequency of Shot Wounds recorded during the War of the Rebellion.

SEAT OF INJURY.	Total Cases.	RESULTS.			Percentage of Fatality.	Relative Frequency
		Recoveries.	Deaths.	Undeterm'd Results.		
Shot Injuries of the Head	12,089	6,573	2,676	2,840	28.9	14.91
Shot Injuries of the Face	9,416	7,406	462	1,548	5.8	10.77 { 3.87
Shot Injuries of the Neck	4,895	3,496	618	781	15.0	1.99
Shot Injuries of the Spine	642	279	349	14	55.5	0.26
Shot Injuries of the Chest	20,264	13,921	5,373	970	27.8	8.24
Shot Injuries of the Abdomen	8,438	3,455	3,293	1,690	48.7	18.37 { 3.43
Shot Injuries of the Pelvis	3,159	2,194	930	35	29.7	1.28
Shot Flesh Wounds of the Back	12,681	10,883	800	998	6.9	5.16
Shot Injuries of the Upper Extremities	87,793	80,090	5,608	2,095	6.5	35.71
Shot Injuries of the Lower Extremities	86,413	73,665	11,813	935	13.8	35.15
Aggregates	245,790	201,962	31,922	11,906	13.6	00.00

Source: Surgical Volume of Part III, The Medical and Surgical History of the War of the Rebellion

Sidelight 9

Monthly reports of sick and wounded, from May 1st, 1861, to June 30th, 1865.

CLASSIFICATION.	WHITE TROOPS.		COLORED TROOPS.		TOTAL.	
	Cases.	Deaths.	Cases.	Deaths.	Cases.	Deaths.
1 Burns	9,487	94	613	4	10,100	98
2 Contusions	44,323	161	2,649	11	46,972	172
3 Concussion of Brain	873	193	49	22	922	215
4 Compression of Brain**	61	17	....	....	61	17
5 Drowning	....	672	....	125	....	797
6 Sprains	38,387	3	4,317	....	42,704	3
7 Dislocations	2,908	9	108	1	3,016	10
8 Fractures	1,287	53	....	....	1,287	53
9 Simple Fractures	4,215	61	131	15	4,346	76
10 Compound Fractures	1,316	378	55	19	1,371	397
11 Gunshot Wounds	229,119	32,731	6,466	922	235,585	33,653
12 Incised Wounds	21,444	186	1,305	3	22,749	189
13 Lacerated Wounds	14,153	459	595	8	14,748	467
14 Puncture Wounds	5,285	191	499	8	5,784	199
15 Poisoning	3,087	93	67	17	3,154	110
16 Other Accidents and Injuries	13,099	1,003	2,174	72	15,273	1,075
Aggregates	389,044	36,304	19,028	1,227	408,072	37,531

**After June 30th, 1863, this class was omitted, as it was found that depressed fractures of the skull were sometimes omitted.

Source: Medical Volume of Part I, The Medical and Surgical History of the War of the Rebellion

CASUALTIES IN MAJOR BATTLES*

	Federal	Confederate
First Bull Run, Va. (July 21, 1861)	2,645	1,981
Fort Donelson, Tenn. (February 12-16, 1862)	2,832	16,623
Shiloh, Tenn. (April 6-7, 1862)	13,047	10,694
Fair Oaks or Seven Pines, Va. (May 31-June 1, 1862)	5,031	6,134
Seven Days' Battle, Va. Peninsular Campaign (June 25-July 1, 1862)	15,849	17,136
Second Bull Run, Va. (August 29-30, 1862)	14,754	8,397
Harper's Ferry, W. Va. (September 12-15, 1862)	11,783	500
Antietam (Sharpsburg), Md. (Sept. 17, 1862)	12,410	13,724
Perryville, Ky. (October 8, 1862)	4,211	3,396
Fredericksburg, Va. (December 13, 1862)	12,653	5,309
Murfreesboro or Stone's River, Tenn. (December 1, 1862-January 2, 1863)	12,906	11,739
Chancellorsville, Va. (May 1-5, 1863)	16,792	12,764
Siege of Vicksburg, Miss. (May 18-July 4, 1863	8,873	39,491
Gettysburg, Pa. (July 1-3, 1863)		
Engaged	88,298	75,000
Killed	3,155	3,903
Wounded	14,529	18,735
Missing	5,365	5,425
Total Losses	23,049	28,063
Chickamauga, Ga. (September 10-21, 1863)	16,170	18,454
Chatanooga Engagements (Tenn.) (November 23-25, 1863)	5,824	6,667
The Wilderness, Va. (May 5-7, 1864)	17,666	7,750
Spotsylvania Court House, Va. (May 8-20, 1864)	18,399	7,750
Cold Harbor, Va. (June 1-3, 1864)	12,000	unknown
Siege of Petersburg, Va. (June 10-April 2, 1864)	42,000	28,000
Atlanta, Ga. (July 22, 1864)	3,722	8,500
Sayler's Creek, VA. (April 6, 1865)	1,180	7,000

Medical and Surgical History of the War of the Rebellion—(1870-1888)
Miller, *Photo History of the Civil War*—1911
National Gallery of Art, *The Civil War*—1961
Eaton, *Original Photographs of the Civil War*—1907
Steiner, *Disease in the Civil War*—1968
Cunningham, *Doctors in Gray*—1958
Adams, *Doctors in Blue*—1952
Steiner, *Medical-Military Portraits*—1968
Confederate States Army, *Manual of Military Surgery*—1863
Medical Society of Virginia, *Confederate Medicine*—1961
Steiner, *Physicians General in the Civil War*—1966
*Livermore. *Numbers and Losses in the Civil War*—1900

Source: "Medicine of the Civil War" booklet published by the National Library of Medicine

Copy

War Department
Surgeon General's Office
Washington City   May 1864

Mr. L. Casella
  No. 23 Halton Garden
    London. England.

Sir:

  I have the honor to inform you that Medical Officers of the U.S. Army are in future to be furnished by the Government with Clinical Thermometers, and to enquire whether you can furnish them, and if so, what price per hundred.

  The style required is a Maximum Thermometer, graduated to half degrees F, so clearly that quarter degrees can readily be estimated by the eye. The graduation to extend from 85° F to 115°, with sufficient room above for expansion to 125°F. Part of them are desired straight, and part curved.

  It is also desirable that if possible the instrument should not be more than ten inches long in order that it may be as strong and as portable as possible. The whole number required will probably be three hundred and I wish to know how soon you can begin to furnish them.

  I am aware that delay in graduating the tubes after they have been filled is desirable, and I wish the instruments to be of the first class workmanship, accurate and corresponding with each other. I should also like to have a sample of the instrument [sic] which you propose to furnish, or of any modifications which you may think proper, delivered to Mr Wm. Wesley by whom this letter will be presented and who will pay for the same. An early reply is requested.

       By order of the Surgeon General,
        Very respectfully
        Your obt. servt.
       (Signed) John S. Billings
       Bvt. Lt. Col. & Asst. Surg. U.S.A.

Source:
Letter to Mr. L. Casella from John Billings, May, 1864;
Bureau of Medicine; Records of the Adjutant General's Office;
Record Group 94; National Archives; Wash. D.C.

Courtesy of Gretchen Worden, Director, Mutter Museum, Philadelphia

Sidelight 12

The quantity of certain of the supplies purchased and manufactured during the war by the Medical Department of the Army.

ARTICLES.	QUANTITY.	ARTICLES.	QUANTITY.
Acaciae pulvis, in ½-lb. bottles ....oz.	869,070	Corn-starch, in 1-lb. papers.....................lbs.	218,708
Acidum aceticum, in ½-lb. g.s. bottles ....oz.	353,477	Farina, in 1-lb. papers..........................lbs.	251,837
Acidum sulphuricum aromaticum ....oz.	395,708	Gelatine, shred, in ¼-lb. packages ....lbs.	13,067
Acidum tannicum, in 1-oz. bottles ....oz.	83,550	Milk, concentrated, in 1-lb. tins................lbs.	479,014
Acidum tartaricum, in 8-oz. bottles ....oz.	399,977	Porter, in pint bottles ....bottles	1,833,948
Aether fortior, in ½-lb. g.s. bottles and ½-lb. tins .oz.	1,002,045	Tea, black, in tins or original chests ....lbs.	429,695
Aetheris spiritus compositus, in ½-lb. g.s. bottles .oz.	357,372	Tapioca, in tins...............................lbs.	85,226
Aetheris spiritus nitrici, in ½-lb. g.s. bottles .....oz.	1,610,361		
Alcohol fortius, in 32-oz. bottles ....bottles	483,930	**INSTRUMENTS.**	
Ammoniae, liquor, in ½-lb. g.s. bottles ....oz.	1,237,627	Amputating cases..............................no.	360
Argenti nitras, in 1-oz. g.s. bottles ....oz.	42,185	Amputating and trephining cases................no.	235
Argenti nitras fusus, in 1-oz. bottles ....oz.	35,818	Compact field cases............................no.	3,955
Camphora, in 8-oz. bottles ....oz.	924,184	Electro-magnetic machines......................no.	20
Ceratum adipis (simple cerate), in 1-lb. pots...lbs.	210,880	Exsecting cases................................no.	150
Ceratum resinae, in 1-lb. pots ....lbs.	51,049	General operating cases.........................no.	596
Chloroform....................................oz.	1,146,982	Minor operating cases..........................no.	77
Creta preparata, in ½ lb. bottles ....oz.	243,048	Personal instruments ....sets	273
Extractum aconiti radicis fluidum, in ½-lb. bottles .oz.	218,326	Pocket cases...................................no.	12,656
Extractum belladonnae, in 1-oz. pots ....oz.	28,243	Post-mortem cases.............................no.	303
Extractum bucho fluidum, in ½-lb. bottles.......oz.	309,896	Trephining cases...............................no.	213
Extractum chichonae fluidum (with aromatics)...oz	518,957	Tourniquets, field..............................no.	50,214
Extractum colocynthidis compositum, in 8-oz. pots.oz.	188,030	Tourniquets, screw, with pad....................no.	13,974
Extractum conii, in 1-oz. pots..................oz.	13,524	Trusses, inguinal, double........................no.	6,350
Extractum gentianae fluidum, in ½-lb. bottles....oz.	347,173	Trusses, single.................................no.	43,529
Extractum hyoscyami, in 1-oz. pots ....oz.	20,534		
Extractum ipecacuanhae fluidum, in ½-lb. bottles .oz.	313,739	**DRESSINGS, Etc.**	
Extractum nucis vomicae, in 1-oz. pots ....oz.	11,989	Adhesive plaster, 5 yards in a can ....yds.	327,943
Extractum pruni virginianae fluidum, in ½-lb. bottles .oz.	307,323	Cotton bats....................................no.	66,727
Extractum rhei fluidum, in ½-lb. bottles.........oz.	258,009	Cotton wadding ....sheets	73,225
Extractum senegae fluidum, in ½-lb. bottles .....oz.	315,633	Flannel, red, all wool...........................yds.	159,593
Extractum valerianae fluidum, in ½-lb. bottles ...oz.	170,525	Gutta-percha cloth.............................yds.	106,011
Extractum zingiberis fluidum, in ½-lb. bottles ...oz.	506,380	Ichthyocolla plaster, 1 yd. in case ....yds.	224,767
Ferri chloridi tinctura, in ½ lb. g.s. bottles ......oz.	616,474	Lint, patent, linen or flax ....lbs.	147,135
Ferri iodidi syrupus, in ½-lb. g.s. bottles ....oz.	162,614	Lint, picked or scraped, linen ....lbs.	82,754
Ferri et quiniae citras, in 1-oz. bottles ....oz.	50,772	Muslin, bleached, unsized, 1 yd. wide ....yds.	3,512,442
Ferri persulphatis liquor, in 4-oz. g.s. bottles ....oz.	130,997	Oiled muslin, in 4½-yd. pieces...................yds.	72,219
Ferri persulphatis pulvis, in 1-oz. g.s. bottles ....oz.	153,741	Oiled silk, in 4½-yd. pieces......................yds.	91,702
Ferri sulphas, in 4-oz. bottles..................oz.	544,045	Roller bandages, assorted, in a pasteboard box ...doz.	668,817
Ferri pilulae, in 8-oz. pots.....................oz.	277,808		
Hydrargyrum cum creta, in ½ lb. bottles.........oz.	69,278	**BEDDING.**	
Ipecacuanhae pulvis, in ½-lb. bottles ....oz.	328,029	Bed-sacks......................................no.	522,246
Ipecaculanhae et opii pulvis, in ½-lb. bottles ....oz.	447,151	Beds, water, of India rubber.....................no.	1,144
Lini pulvis, in tins ....lbs.	415,996	Blankets, white; gray for the field ....no.	1,165,805
Magnesiae sulphas..............................lbs.	515,828	Counterpanes, according to pattern..............no.	496,759
Morphiae sulphas, in 4-oz. bottles ....oz.	27,200	Cushions, rubber, with open centre ....no.	6,486
Oleum ricini, in 32-oz. bottles ....oz.	220,334	Cushions, rubber for air or water, small..........no.	11,724
Opii pulvis, in ½-lb. bottles ....oz.	552,196	Gutta-percha bed-covers........................no.	39,551
Opii tinctura, in ½-lb. bottles ....oz.	828,258	Mattresses, hair, in two equal parts, to pack folded...no.	75,920
Opii tinctura camphorata, in ½-lb. bottles........oz.	993,311	Mattresses, of straw, moss or shucks.............no.	169,080
Pilulae opii, in g.s. bottles.....................doz.	813,156	Mosquito-bars, when specially required ....no.	221,058
Potassae bitartras, in ½-lb. bottles..............oz.	556,488	Pillows, hair...................................no.	367,513
Potassae chloras, in ½-lb. bottles ....oz.	568,923	Pillow-cases, cotton, colored....................no.	631,801
Potassii iodidum, in ½-lb. bottles ....oz.	531,744	Pillow-cases, linen, white ....no.	418,365
Quiniae sulphas, compressed in 5-oz. tins ....oz.	595,544	Pillow-ticks....................................no.	318,815
Rhei pulvis, in 4-oz. bottles....................oz.	132,552	Sheets, linen ....no.	1,638,770
Scillae syrupus, in 1-lb. bottles.................lbs.	183,582		
Sodae chlorinatae liquor, in 1-lb. g.s. bottles .....lbs.	167,459	**FURNITURE AND APPLIANCES.**	
Sodae bicarbonas, in ½-lb. bottles ....oz.	652,913	Basins, tin, wash-hand ....no.	92,893
Sodae et potasse tartras, in ½-lb. bottles.........oz.	798,553	Bed-pans, delf, shovel-shape....................no.	38,378
Spiritus lavandulae compositus, in ½-lb. bottles...oz.	404,117	Bedsteads, iron................................no.	274,704
Spiritus frumenti (whiskey), in 32-oz. bottles ...bottles	1,907,145	Close-stools...................................no.	9,737
Spiritus vini gallici, in 32-oz. bottles...........bottles	582,187	Lanterns, glass................................no.	39,499
Vinum album (sherry), in 32-oz. bottles..........bottles	736,459	Medicine panniers, furnished by the list..........no.	5,830
Zinci chloridi liquor, in 1-lb. g.s. bottles ....oz.	486,966	Medicine wagons...............................no.	251
Zinci sulphas, in 1-oz. bottles ....oz.	92,805	Mess-chests, furnished by list...................no.	3,954
		Mugs, delf....................................no.	247,993
HOSPITAL STORES.		Pitchers, delf, half-gallon ....no.	35,433
		Pitchers, delf..................................no.	472,022
Arrow root.....................................lbs.	62,226	Rauges, size as required, with fixtures complete...no.	204
Beef, extract of, in 2-lb. tins ....lbs.	570,980	Spittoons......................................no.	89,169
Cocoa, or chocolate, in tins or cakes.............lbs.	129,596	Stoves, cooking, with fixtures complete...........no.	1,821
Coffee, extract of, in ½-gal. tins ....gals.	25,317		

Source: Medical Volume of Part III, Medical and Surgical History of the War of the Rebellion

Sidelight 13

Summary of Sixty Thousand Two Hundred and Sixty-six Shot Fractures of the Extremities, showing Treatment and Results.

MODE OF TREATMENT.	Cases.	Recovery.	Fatal.	Undetermined.	Percentage of Fatality.	UPPER EXTREMITIES				LOWER EXTREMITIES			
						Recovery.	Fatal.	Undetermined.	Percentage of Fatality.	Recovery.	Fatal.	Undetermined.	Percentage of Fatality.
Conservation....................	26,467	20,854	4,562	1,051	17.9	11,646	1,288	480	9.9	9,208	3,274	571	26.2
Excision	4,656	3,183	1,213	260	27.5	2,744	858	239	23.8	439	355	21	44.7
Amputation......................	29,143	20,338	7,086	1,719	25.8	12,539	1,822	1,376	12.6	7,799	5,264	343	40.2
Aggregates	60,266	44,375	12,861	3,030	22.4	26,929	3,968	2,095	12.8	17,446	8,893	935	33.7

Source: Surgical Volumes of Part III, The Medical and Surgical History of the War of the Rebellion

Sidelight 14

GENERAL ORDERS } No. 158

WAR DEPARTMENT,
ADJUTANT GENERAL'S OFFICE,
Washington, May 29, 1863

The following uniform has been adopted for officers of the Invalid Corps:

Frock Coat—Of sky-blue cloth, with dark-blue velvet collar and cuffs—in all other respects, according to the present pattern for officers of Infantry.

Shoulder Straps—According to present regulations, but worked on dark-blue velvet.

Pantaloons—Of sky-blue cloth, with double stripe of dark-blue cloth down the outer seam, each stripe one-half inch wide, with space between of three-eighths of an inch.

BY ORDER OF THE SECRETARY OF WAR:

E. D. TOWNSEND
Assistant Adjutant General

GENERAL ORDERS } No. 124

WAR DEPARTMENT,
ADJUTANT GENERAL'S OFFICE,
Washington, May 15, 1863

The following uniform has been adopted for the Invalid Corps:

Jacket—Of sky-blue kersey, with dark-blue trimmings, cut like the jacket for United States cavalry, to come well down on the loins and abdomen.

Trowsers—Present regulation, sky-blue.

Forage Cap—Present regulation.

BY ORDER OF THE SECRETARY OF WAR:

E. D. TOWNSEND
Assistant Adjutant General

Sidelight 15

ENLISTMENTS AND DEATHS
ENLISTMENTS*

Union 2,893,304
Confederacy somewhere between 1,277,890 and 1,406,180

DEATHS

Union*
  In battle 110,070
  Disease 224,586
  Accidents, suicides, etc. 24,872
    Total 359,528

Confederacy*
  In battle 94,000
  Disease, etc. 164,000
    Total 258,000
Total, Union and Confederacy 617,528

*Reducing these figures to the standard of three-year enlistments, Livermore put Union strength at 1,556,678 and confederate strength at 1,082,119.
**Adjutant General's Officer (1885).
***Burke.

Source:"Medicine of the Civil War" booklet published by the National Library of Medicine

Sidelight 16

WOUNDS AND SICKNESS (Union)*

Wounds

Of the 246,712 cases of wounds reported in the Medical Records by weapons of war, 245,790 were shot wounds and 922 were sabre and bayonet.

Sickness

Of 5,825,480 admissions to sick report there were:

Cases		Deaths
75,368	typhoid	27,050
2,501	typhus	850
11,898	continued fever	147
49,871	typho-malarial fever	4,059
1,155,266	acute diarrhea	2,923
170,488	chronic diarrhea	27,558
233,812	acute dysentery	4,084
25,670	chronic dysentery	3,229
73,382	syphilis	123
95,833	gonorrhea	6
30,714	scurvy	383
3,744	delirium tremens	450
2,410	insanity	80
2,837	paralysis	231

*Official Records

Source: "Medicine of the Civil War" booklet published by the National Library of Medicine

Sidelight 17

About 1, P.M., spasmodic contractions of the muscles came on, causing pronation of the forearms; the pectoral muscles seemed to be fixed, the breath was held during the spasm, and a sudden and forcible expiration immediately succeeded it.

At about the same time both pupils became widely dilated, and remained so until death.

During the night Drs. HALL, MAY, LIEBERMANN, and nearly all the leading men of the profession in the city, tendered their services.

AUTOPSY; FIVE HOURS AFTER DEATH

Present, Surgeon-General BARNES, Col. CRANE, Dr. STONE, Ass't Surg. WOODWARD, U.S.A. Ass't Surg. CURTIS, U.S.A. Ass't Surg. NOTSON, U.S.A., and Act'g Ass't Surg. TAFT, U.S.A.

The calvaria was removed, the brain exposed, and sliced down to the track of the ball, which was plainly indicated by a line of coagulated blood, extending from the external wound in the occipital bone, obliquely across from the left to right through the brain to the anterior lobe of the cerebrum, immediately behind the right orbit. The surface of the right hemisphere was covered with coagulated blood. After removing the brain from the cranium, the ball dropped from its lodgment in the anterior lobe. A small piece of the ball evidently cut off in its passage through the occipital bone, was previously taken out of the track of the ball, about four inches from the external wound. The hole made through the occipital bone was as cleanly cut as if done with a punch.

The point of entrance was one inch to the left of the longitudinal sinus, and opening into the lateral sinus. The ball was flattened, convex on both sides, and evidently moulded by hand in a Derringer pistol mould, as indicated by the ridged surface left by the nippers in clipping off the neck.

The orbital plates of *both* orbits were the seats of comminuted fracture, the fragments being forced inward, and the dura-mater covering them remaining uninjured. The double fracture was decided to have been caused by *contre coup*. The plug of bone driven in from the occipital bone was found in the track of the ball, about three inches from the external wound, proving the correctness of the opinion advanced by the Surgeon-General and Dr. Stone as to its nature, at the exploration of the wound before death.

The ball and fragments, together with the fragments of the orbital plates and plug from the occipital bone, were placed in the possession of Dr. Stone, the family physician, who marked and delivered them, pursuant to instructions, to the Secretary of State, who sealed them up with his private seal. The *Nelaton* probe used was also marked by me, and sealed up in like manner.

Medical and Surgical Reporter Philadelphia April 22, 1865
"The Last Hours of Abraham Lincoln"
By C.S. Taft, Act'g Ass't Surg. U.S.A.

Courtesy of Gretchen Worden, Director, Mutter Museum, Philadelphia

Bibliography

American Armamentarium Chirurgicum. 1889. Reprint, San Francisco: Norman Publishing & Printers Devil, 1989.

Armed Forces Institute of Pathology. *The Billings Microscope Collection.* 2d ed. Washington, D.C., 1980.

Ashburn, P. M. *A History of the Medical Department of the United States Army.* Boston: Houghton Mifflin: 1929.

Ballou, Charles F., III, M.D. "Confederate Medicine: Civil War Doctors on the Brink of a New Era in Medicine." *Tufts Medicine* (Summer 1995): 17-24.

Barnes, Joseph K. et al. ed., *The Medical and Surgical History of the War of the Rebellion, 1861-1865.* 12 vols. Washington, D.C.: GPO, 1870-88.

Bettmann, Otto L. *A Pictorial History of Medicine.* Springfield, Ill.: Charles C. Thomas, 1956.

Billings, John D., and Charles W. Reed. *Hardtack and Coffee.* 1887. Reprint, N.p.: University of Nebraska Press, 1993.

Blanton, Wyndham B. *Medicine in Virginia in the Nineteenth Century.* Richmond, 1933.

Blochman, Lawrence G. *Doctor Squibb: the Life and Times of a Rugged Idealist.* New York: Simon and Schuster, 1958.

Bollet, Alfred Jay, M.D. "To Care for Him That has Borne the Battle." Parts 1 and 2. *Medical Times* 118, no. 5 (April 1989); 118, no. 6 (June 1990): 39-44.

Boyden, Anna L. *Echoes From Hospital and White House.* Boston: D. Lothrop and Company, 1884.

Browning, William, M.D. "The Case of Instruments Used at the Autopsy, April 15, 1865, on the Body of President Lincoln." *Medical Times* (September 1935): 282-83. Courtesy Gretchen Worden, Director, Mutter Museum, Philadelphia

Bullock and Crenshaw. *Catalogue of Drugs, Medicines, Utensils, Surgical Instruments, etc.* Philadelphia, 1857.

Childs, Timothy, M.D. "Objections to Exclusive Systems in Medicine." *American Medical Monthly* 7 (May 1857): 275.

Chisolm, J. Julian. *Manual of Military Surgery for the Use of Surgeons in the Confederate States Army.* 3rd ed. Columbia, 1864.

Civil War Through the Eyes of the Camera, The. Springfield, Mass.: Patriot Publishing, 1912.

Damman, Gordon. *Pictorial Encyclopedia of Civil War Medical Instruments and Equipment.* 2 vols. Missoula, Mont.: Pictorial Histories Publishing Company, 1984-94.

Dannett, Sylvia G. L., comp. ed. *Noble Women of the North.* New York: Thomas Yoseloff, 1959.

Denny, Robert E. *Civil War Medicine: Care & Comfort of the Wounded.* New York: Sterling, 1994.

"Doctors Debate Cause of Lincoln's Death." *The Civil War General News* (April 1995): 22. Courtesy Gretchen Worden, Director, Mutter Museum, Philadelphia.

Druitt, Robert, M.D. *The Principles and Practice of Modern Surgery.* Rev. ed. Philadelphia: Blanchard and Lea, 1860.

Duffy, John. *The Healers: The Rise of the Medical Establishment.* New York: McGraw-Hill, 1976.

Dulles, Foster Rhea. *The American Red Cross.* New York: Harper & Brothers, 1950.

Duncan, Louis C. *The Medical Department of the United States Army in the Civil War.* Reprint, Gaithersburg: Olde Soldier Books, n.d.

Edmonds, S. Emma. *Nurse and Spy.* Hartford: W.S. Williams; Philadelphia: Jones Bros., 1865.

Ellis, Thomas T., M.D. *Leaves From the Diary of an Army Surgeon: or, Incidents of Field Camp, and Hospital Life.* New York: John Bradburn, 1863.

Engle, Eloise. *Medic: America's Medical Soldiers, Sailors and Airmen in Peace and War.* New York: John Day Company, 1967.

Flint, Austin, M.D. *A Treatise on the Principles and Practice of Medicine.* 2d ed., rev. Philadelphia: Henry C. Lea, 1867.

Foster, Frank P., M.D. *An Illustrated Encyclopaedic Medical Dictionary.* 4 vols. New York: D. Appleton and Company, 1892.

Garrison, Fielding H., M.D. *An Introduction to the History of Medicine,* 3rd ed. Philadelphia: W.B. Saunders Company, 1924.

Goodrich, Frank B. *The Tribute Book: A Record of the Munificence, Self-Sacrifice and Patriotism of the American People During the War for the Union.* New York: Derby & Miller, 1865.

Greenbie, Marjorie Barstow. *Lincoln's Daughters of Mercy.* New York: G.P. Putnam's Sons, 1944.

Gross, Samuel D., M.D. *Systems of Surgery.* Vol. I. Philadelphia: Blanchard & Lea, 1862.

Gunn, John C., M.D. *Gunn's New Family Physician: or Home Book of Health.* 100th ed., rev. and enl. New York: Moore, Wilstach & Baldwin, 1865.

Hambrecht, F. Terry, M.D., M. Rhode, and A. Hawk. "Dr. Chisolm's Inhaler: A Rare Confederate Medical Invention." *The Journal of South Carolina Association,* (May 1991): 277-80.

Hogg, Jabez. *The Microscope: Its History, Construction, and Application.* London: Routledge, Warne, and Routledge, 1861.

Hornung, Clarence P., ed. *Handbook of Early Advertising Art.* 3rd ed. New York: Dover Publications, 1956.

Hume, Edgar Erskine. *Victories of Army Medicine.* Philadelphia: J.B. Lippincott Company, 1943.

Hurd, Charles. *The Compact History of the American Red Cross.* New York: Hawthorn Books, 1957.

———. *Instrumentalities for Surgery, Therapeutics and Biology.* 7th ed. New York: John Reynders, 1895.

James, Edward T., and Janet James, ed. *Notable American Women 1607-1950: A Biographical Dictionary.* 3 vols. Cambridge, Mass.: Belknap Press of Harvard University, 1973.

Keen W. W., M.D. "The Contrast Between the Surgery of the Civil War and That of the Present War." *New York Medical Journal* (April 1915): 1–25.

———. *Military Surgery in 1861 and in 1918: The Annals of American Academy of Political and Social Science.* Philadelphia, 1918.

Klawans, Harold L. "Court-Martial of a Surgeon." *M. D.* (April 1992): 103–6, 109, 113–15.

Knight, Nancy. "Pain and Its Relief." From an Exhibition of the National Museum of History. Smithsonian Institution, 1986.

LeGrand, Louis, M.D. *The Military Hand-Book and Soldier's Manual of Information.* 1861. Reprint, Jacksonville, Ill.: C.W. Heritage, n.d.

Livermore, Mary A. *My Story of the War: A Woman's Narrative of Four Years Personal Experience.* Hartford: A.D. Worthington and Company, 1888.

Lord, Francis A. *Civil War Collector's Encyclopedia.* Harrisburg, Penn.: Stackpole Company, 1963.

Major, Ralph H., M.D. *A History of Medicine.* Vol. 2. Springfield, Ill.: Charles C. Thomas, 1954.

Margotta, Roberto. *The Story of Medicine.* ed. Paul Louis. New York: Golden Press, 1968.

Maxwell, William Quentin. *Lincoln's Fifth Wheel: The Politcal History of the United States Sanitary Commission.* New York: Longmans, Green & Co., 1956.

McCarthy, Carlton. *Soldier Life in the Confederate Army.* N.p., 1882.

Medicine of the Civil War. The National Library of Medicine, n.d.

Mitchell, Thomas D., M.D. *Materia Medica and Therapeutics: with Ample Illustration of Practice.* Philadelphia: Lippincott and Co., 1857.

Moore, Frank. *Women of the War: Their Heroism and Self-Sacrifice.* Hartford: S.S. Scranton & Co., 1866.

"Murder of President Lincoln." *Medical and Surgical Reporter* 12 (April 1865): 452. Courtesy Gretchen Worden, Director, Mutter Museum, Philadelphia.

Nightingale, Florence. *Notes on Nursing: What It Is, And What It Is Not.* New York: D. Appleton and Company, 1860.

Olmsted, Frederick Law. *Hospital Transport: A Memoir of the Embarkation of the Sick and Wounded from the Peninsula of Virginia in the Summer of 1862.* Boston: Ticknor and Fields, 1863.

Packard, Francis R., M.D. *History of Medicine in the United States.* 2 vols. New York: Paul B. Hoeber, 1931.

Padgitt, Donald L. *A Short History of the Early American Microscope.* London, Microscope Publications Ltd., 1975.

Philadelphia Museum of Art. *Medicine and the Artist.* 3rd ed., enl. New York: Dover Publications, 1970.

Pollard, Edward A. *The First Year of the War.* Richmond: West & Johnston, 1862.

———. *The Lost Cause: A New Southern History of the War of the Confederates.* New York: E.B. Treat & Co., 1866.

Rosenberg, Charles E. *The Care of Strangers.* New York: Basic Books, 1987.

Ross, Ishbel. *Child of Destiny: The Life Story of the First Woman Doctor.* New York: Harper & Brothers, 1949.

Soldier Life in the Union and Confederate Armies. Ed. Philip Van Doren Stern. Bloomington, Ind.: Indiana University Press, 1961.

Syme, James. *Principles and Practice of Surgery.* ed. Robert S. Newton, M.D. Cincinnati: E. Morgan & Co., 1857.

Taft, C.S. "Last Hours of Abraham Lincoln." *Medical and Surgical Reporter* 12 (April 1865): 452–54. Courtesy Gretchen Worden, Director, Mutter Museum, Philadelphia.

Tormey, David M. "Infectious Disease Was Far Costlier For Soldiers than Bloody Battle." *Hall A.* 12 (Spring 1995): 42–44.

Truesdale, John. *The Blue Coats: and How They Lived, Fought and Died for the Union.* Philadelphia: Jones Brothers & Co., 1867.

Wales, Philip S., M.D. *Elementary Operations in Surgery.* Philadelphia: Henry C. Lea, 1867.

Walter, Richard D. "William Hammond and His Enemies." *Bulletin of the Los Angeles Neurological Society,* (1968): 322–31.

Wiley, Bell Irvin. *The Life of Johnny Reb: the Common Soldier of the Confederacy.* Indianapolis: Bobbs–Merrill Company, 1943.

Wood, George B., M.D. *A Treatise on the Practice of Medicine.* 5th ed. 2 vols. Philadelphia: J.B. Lippincott and Co., 1858.

Wood, George W., M.D., and Franklin Bache, M.D. *The Dispensatory of the United States of America.* 8th ed. rev. Philadelphia: Grigg, Elliot, and Co., 1849.

Wormeley, Katharine Prescott. *The Other Side of the War With the Army of the Potomac.* Boston: Ticknor and Company, 1889.

Young, Agatha. *The Women and the Crisis: Women of the North in the Civil War.* New York: McDowell, Obolensky, 1959.

U.S. Department of Agriculture. *Mosquitoes of Medical Importance.* Agriculture Handbook No. 152. Washington, D.C.: GPO, 1959.

U.S. Surgeon General. *A Manual of Military Surgery.* Prepared for the Use of the Confederate States Army. Richmond: Ayres & Wade, Illustrated News Steam Presses, 1863.

———. *Military Sanitation and First Aid.* Washington, D.C.: GPO, 1940.

———. *The Medical and Surgical History of the War of the Rebellion.* 2 vols. Washington, D.C.: GPO, 1870–83.

Picture Credits

R=Right
L=Left
▲=top
◆=center
▼=bottom
Page locations
AAC=Tiemann, *The American Armamentarium Chirurgicum* 1898
MSHR=*Medical and Surgical History of the War of the Rebellion* pub. 1870-1888
Reynders dates - 1883 pic copyright, 1895 publ. date

	R▼	*MSHR*
30	All	Billings, *Soldier Life in the Union Army,* 1887
31	R▲(all)	Author's sketches, Gettysburg National Military Museum
32	L♦	Author's sketch, Gettysburg National Military Museum
	R♦	Author's sketch, Civil War Museum, Philadelphia
33	L▲	Author's sketch, Gettysburg National Military Museum
	R▲	Author's sketch, Gettysburg National Military Museum
	R▼	Author's sketch, Gettysburg National Military Museum
34	R▲	Hume, *Victories of Army Medicine,* 1943
35	R▲	*MSHR*
	L▲	*MSHR*
36	R▲	Author's sketch
	L▼	Author's sketch
37	All	*MSHR*
38	▲5 illus	*MSHR*
	▼	(confederate stretcher) Chisolm, *A Manual of Military Surgery,* 1864
39	▼	Druitt, *The Principles and Practice of Modern Surgery,* 1860
40	L+R▲	Druitt, *The Principles and Practice of Modern Surgery,* 1860
	R▲	(Bandage roller) Foster, *An Illustrated Medical Dictionary,* 1892
	L▼♦	Druitt, *The Principles and Practice of Modern Surgery,* 1852
	L▼	*MSHR*
41	L▼♦R▼	*MSHR*
42	L+R▼	"Harper's Weekly," New York, 1862
43	R♦	Author's retouched photo
	R▼	Author's sketch
44	L▲	Tiemann, *AAC,* 1889
	R♦	Knight, *Pain and Its Relief,* Smithsonian Institution
	L▼	(A period rag doll) *Index of American Design,* National Gallery of Art, Washington, D.C.
45	L▲	*MSHR*
	R▲	New York Academy of Medicine
	L♦	Author's sketch
	R▼	*MSHR*
46	L▲	*MSHR*
	R♦	Gross, *Systems of Surgery,* Vol. I, 1862
47	R♦	Reynders, *Instrumentalities,* 1883 (1895)
	L▼	Ashhurst, *International Encyclopedia,* 1881
	R▼	Wilbur, *Antique Medical Instruments,* Third Edition, 1998
	R▼	Tiemann, *AAC,* 1889
48	Top	Tiemann, *AAC,* 1889; Reynders, *Instrumentalities,* 1883 (1895); Wales, *Elementary Operations,* 1867; Druitt, *The Principles and Practice of Modern Surgery,* 1860; Gross, *Systems of Surgery,* Vol. I, 1862; Tiemann, *AAC,* 1889
	Bottom	Druitt, *The Principles and Practice of Modern Surgery,* Vol. I, 1862
	R▼	Gross, *Systems of Surgery* Vol. I, 1862
49	R▲	Druitt, *The Principles and Practice of Modern Surgery,* Vol. I, 1862
	R▼	Author's sketch, Gettysburg National Military Museum
50	R▲	Dannett, *Noble Women of the North,* 1959
	R♦	Tiemann, *AAC,* 1889
	L▼	Author's sketch, Gettysburg National Military Museum
51	R▲▼♦	Tiemann, *AAC,* 1889; Gross, *Systems of Surgery,* Vol. I, 1862
52	L▲	Reynders, *Instrumentalities,* 1883 (1895); Druitt, *The Principles and Practice of Modern Surgery*
	L▼	Tiemann, *AAC,* 1889
	R▼	Druitt, *The Principles and Practice of Modern Surgery,* Vol. I, 1860
53	Top	Various period medical and instrument catalogs
	L▼♦	Druitt, *The Principles and Practice of Modern Surgery,* Vol. I, 1862
54	L▲	Reynders, *Instrumentalities,* 1883 (1895)
	L▼♦	Druitt, *The Principles and Practice of Modern Surgery,* Vol. I, 1862
55	R▲	Druitt, *The Principles and Practice of Modern Surgery,* Vol. I, 1860
	R	Reynders, *Instrumentalities,* 1883 (1895)
56	L▲	Reynders, *Instrumentalities,* 1883 (1895)
	R♦	Druitt, *The Principles and Practice of Modern Surgery,* Vol. I, 1860
57	R▲	*MSHR*
	L+R♦	*MSHR*
	R▼	Dannett, *Noble Women of the North,* 1959
58	L+R▼▲♦	Author's sketch
59	L+R♦	*MSHR*
60	R▲	Goodrich, *The Tribute Book,* 1865
	R+L▼	*MSHR*
61	R+L▲	Goodrich, *The Tribute Book,* 1865
	R+L▼	*MSHR*

62	R▲	Livermore, *My Story of the War,* 1888
	L▼	*MSHR*
63	R♦	Author's sketch
	R▼	Dannett, *Noble Women of the North,* 1959
64	R+L▲♦	1) Reynders, *Instrumentalities,* 1883 (1895)
		2) Tiemann, *AAC,* 1889
		3) Reynders, *Instrumentalities,* 1883 (1895)
		4) Reynders, *Instrumentalities,* 1883 (1895)
		5) Tiemann, *AAC,* 1889
		6) Druitt, *The Principles and Practice of Modern Surgery,* 1860
		7) Wilbur, *Antique Medical Instruments,* Third Edition, 1998
		8) Padgitt, *A Short History of the Early American Microscopes,* 1975
65	L▲	Author's sketch, Museum of Royal College of Surgeons, London
	R▲	Author's sketch, Wellcome Historical Medical Museum, London
	L♦	Newton, *Principles and Practice of Surgery,* 1857
	R♦	Hogg, *The Microscope,* Fifth Edition, London, New York, 1861
	L+R▼	Druitt, *The Principles and Practice of Modern Surgery,* 1860
	R▼	Author's sketch of period tooth key—his collection
66	R♦	Druitt, *The Principles and Practice of Modern Surgery,* 1860
	L▼	Reynders, *Instrumentalities,* 1883 (1895)
67	R▲	Ashhurst, *Medical Dictionary,* 1881
	R♦	2 forceps, Tiemann, *AAC,* 1889
	R▼	Druitt, *The Principles and Practice of Modern Surgery,* 1860
68	Full plate	*MSHR*
69	Top	Reynders, *Instrumentalities,* 1883 (1895)
	R+L▼	Author's sketch, National Museum of Civil War Medicine, Frederick, MD
70	R+L♦	Wilbur, *Revolutionary Medicine* 1700-1800, Second Edition, 1997
	R▼	Chisolm, *Manual of Military Surgery,* (Confederate States Army), 1864
	R♦	Foster, *Illustrated Medical Dictionary,* 1892
		Druitt, *The Principles and Practice of Modern Surgery,* 1860
71	L▲	*MSHR*
	L♦	Tiemann, *AAC,* 1889 and Reynders, *Instrumentalities,* 1883 (1895), instrument catalogues
72	R♦	*MSHR*
	L▼	Hume, *Victories of Army Medicine,* 1943
73	R▲	*MSHR*
74	R▲	Author's sketch
	R▼	Goodrich, *The Tribute Book,* 1865
75	L▼	Author's sketch
	R▼	Goodrich, *The Tribute Book,* 1865
76	R♦	Dannett, *Noble Women of the North,* 1959
77	L▲	Moore, *Women of the War,* 1866
	R▼	Moore, *Women of the War,* 1866
78	R▲	Moore, *Women of the War,* 1866
	L♦	Moore, *Women of the War,* 1866
	R▼	Moore, *Women of the War,* 1866
79	L▲	*The World Book Encyclopedia,* 1958
	R▼	Moore, *Women of the War,* 1866
80	L+R▲	Livermore, *My Story of the War,* 1888
81	R▲	Hogg, *The Microscope,* 1860
	R▼	Author's sketch
82	R▼▲	"Bullock & Crenshaw Catalogue," 1857
83	R▲	*Military Sanitation and First Aid,* 1940
	R♦	*Military Sanitation and First Aid,* 1940
84	R▲	Druitt, *The Principles and Practice of Modern Surgery,* 1860
	L♦	Reynders, *Instrumentalities,* 1883 (1895)
85	R▲	Druitt, *The Principles and Practice of Modern Surgery,* 1860
	L▼	*MSHR*
86	L▲	Billings, *Soldier Life in the Union Army,* 1887
87	R▲	Foster, *An Illustrated Encyclopaedic Medical Dictionary,* 1892
	R+L♦	*MSHR*
88	Full page	"Bullock & Crenshaw Catalogue," 1857
89	Full page	"Bullock & Crenshaw Catalogue," 1857
90	L▼	Goodrich, *The Tribute Book,* 1865
91	R▼▲	Parrish, *Treatise on Pharmacy,* 3rd ed., 1867
92	L▼	Parrish, *Treatise on Pharmacy,* 3rd ed., 1867
93	R▲	Foster, *An Illustrated Encyclopaedic Medical Dictionary,* 1892
	L+R▼	"American Druggists' Circular and Chemical Gazette," March 1862
94	Full page	"Bullock & Crenshaw Catalogue," 1857
95	L+R▲♦	"Bullock & Crenshaw Catalogue," 1857

96	L▲	Civil War period, New York newspaper clipping
	L+R▼	Leath & Ross, Homeopathic Chemists & Medical publishers, (broadside), 1861
97	R+L◆	"Gunn's Medical Flora," 1865 (in *Gunn's Family Physician*)
98	R▲	"Civil War General News Special Issue," (clipping) (ND)
99	R◆	Artist was W.W. Cheyne, London, 1892 (clipping)
100	R+L◆	Hornung, *Handbook of Early Advertising Art,* Third Edition, 1956

Index

Italicized items are illustrations.